Praise for *You Can't Judge a Body by Its Cover*...

"We should be taught from the beginning that we are housed in the most beautiful technology on earth, regardless of skin hue. This necessary, crucial book helps women notice what they *truly want*, which is key in the body and weight journey."
—Dr. Alauna Curry, Trauma Psychiatrist, creator of Empathy Skills Practice™ for Traumatized Humans and founder of the Dr. Alauna Trauma Recovery Institute, U.S.

"Chronic shame and self-disgust is a nightmare. This book's perspective helps me to wake up from that nightmare into the new, gentler, deeply compassionate, honoring world Bedrick is cultivating. I wish for everyone to have a taste of this world."
—Esther Dee, U.S.

"Bedrick is a process-oriented psychotherapist with a profound respect for the deep intelligence embedded in women's body experiences. His understanding of the impact of sexism, female socialization, and internalized oppression on the emotional and physical health and wellness of women is palpable on every page and woven through every story."
—Jan Dworkin, PhD, psychologist and author of *Make Love Better: How to Own Your Story, Connect with Your Partner, and Deepen Your Relationship Practice*, U.S.

"With deep compassion, precise awareness, and great skills, Bedrick elicits what is truly behind women's "failure" around dieting. These stories show that women are actually attempting to free themselves from the cage made by the cultural hypnosis and live their own power, beauty, and wisdom.

I see my friends, my clients, and myself in these stories. I wish this book had been available in my teens and twenties, when I felt ashamed of my body and made a number of attempts to lose weight. Nevertheless, this book has brought deep healing to the ashamed part in me and given me new awareness of how better I could help and empower others in their journey to become who they really are."

—Ayako "Aya" Fujisaki, PhD, LPC, U.S.

"What ties all these stories together is the quiet violence perpetuated on our bodies and psyches due to cultural bias and conditioning, however insidious, and the visible and invisible marks these leave on us. You will be left with a feeling of connectedness—of "I am not alone in this"—and an overwhelming sense of love."

—Ernestine Kontogianni, South Africa

"The author's compassionate gaze shines through every page, as this book takes me beyond what is deemed the appropriate health-and-body-weight conversation to where the deepest desires and self-knowing inside our bodies is wanting us truly to go: into the long-ignored, inconvenient, non-commodifiable but ultimately transcendent conversation."

—Jill Hileman, U.S.

"I never saw an overweight woman in any of these stories. I saw again and again a wonderful and beautiful soul. In every single story, these shared insights that touched me, made me reflect. I felt a lot of sympathy (tears flowed!) and happiness for these women."

—Gertrud Kessler, coach, facilitator, and
organizational developer, Switzerland

"I am one and all of these women in varying degrees and I, through reading this important work, have embraced Bedrick's witness to my and other women's struggle for the freedom to feel validated and live authentically."

—Wanda Garcia, M.Ed., U.S.

"Bedrick brings a combination of objective witnessing and conscious compassion in his assessments of the women's experiences by reframing their perceptions of inherent weakness to notice strengths in how they coped with some daunting challenges. Many women uncovered examples of shame, misplaced blame and abuses that had resulted in symptoms related to depression and anxiety due to extremely critical views about how they look.

You Can't Judge a Body by Its Cover offers details of Bedrick's empathic interventions and broad perspectives by taking into account that while body weight is a shallow indicator, realistic options for empowerment can be honed when individuals see themselves more holistically by recognizing political, cultural, and social factors that affect human lives across diverse groups."

—Fannie LeFlore, M.S., psychotherapist and developer of
Healing from Racism Programs, U.S.

"This book is "killing me softly" with these women's songs, but I figure one has to die over and over, to be born again and again.

This book has all the properties and potency of long rushing waters, most distinctively its ability to wear away at the mineralized patriarchal constructs of thinness as the perfect female body, the focus on which insidiously leaches the life force out of so many women, sometimes for their whole lives!"

—Leonora Lorenzo, LCSW, psychotherapist, U.S.

"While reading the stories of these women and their struggles to find the deeper truths about why their bodies had grown bigger as they felt powerless in so many other areas of their lives, I began to quickly sense these same truths for myself. It's an arrow into consciousness. This book is saving my life."

—Andrea Morris MSW, LCSW, psychotherapist, U.S.

"In this book, we learn that shame, despite its proclivity for destruction, has hidden secrets. Wisdom can be found in its shadows.

Bedrick masterfully allows the women to relax into a safe space and get in touch with long-forgotten parts of themselves that lived in the shadow of shame. He follows signals that lead women towards creating an authentic and congruent self. He also allows these women to inform, educate, and transform him. The privilege of witnessing this process through the narratives is the brilliance of this book."

—Rita Mesch, psychologist, Australia Centre for Psychotherapy, Australia

"When I read this book, it was as if Bedrick were talking directly to me, making such powerful and real material not only accessible and engaging, but safe to reflect upon. I found myself asking questions of my own journey with my body, weight, and food. I've come away from each chapter with either an affirmation of a place where I stand now, or encouragement to shine light in areas I've been unwilling to illuminate in the past."

—Carolyn MacLaury, M.Div., End of Life Doula, U.S.

"David Bedrick's new book, *You Can't Judge a Body by Its Cover*, is one of the most exciting, insightful books I've read in a long time. After working one-on-one with many women who struggle not only with their weight but with internalized assaults, criticism, and the viewpoint that something is wrong with them, he has written a masterpiece that dismantles the shame fortress and helps us connect with our deeper body intelligence."

—Crystal Andrus Morissette, author of *The Emotional Edge*, CEO of SWAT (Simply Woman Accredited Trainer) Institute, Canada

"This book is like a series of detective stories! Some stories touched me deeply and brought tears to my eyes, but the more I read, the more an overwhelming sense of calmness appeared. While my mind was busy discovering exciting stories, little by little, effortlessly, a deeper part of myself was undergoing transformation."

—Aleksandra Raczyńska, psychotherapist and business owner, Poland

"In a world of quick fixes, *You Can't Judge a Body by Its Cover* is a breath of fresh air that invites true self-mastery, authenticity, and an opportunity to occupy oneself.

Bedrick's true lack of judgement is a rare gem. In this book, he teases out the authentic process of each individual, and discovers the meaning behind each individual's process. His curiosity, commitment, and passion to discover what wants to reveal itself in each case study is fascinating, while helping me to reflect on my own process. Not only will this book help me have compassion for my students and in my work, it will help me have compassion for myself, my body, and my judgement about my own life process."

—**Kelle Rae Oien, Nia Somatic Education faculty, StudioNia Santa Fe, co-owner and rolfer of Structural Integration, U.S.**

"When I began to read the book, I was not expecting the plethora of emotions that would surge from within me. I moved through electrifying feelings of anger, sadness, compassion, grief, and gratitude. I saw aspects of myself in each of the stories. I experienced an eating disorder from my early teens to early thirties. When I read this book, a raw vulnerability, understanding and compassion ensued. It's as though for the first time I was seen and safely held.

This book is a gift to humanity. Bedrick's loving, patient, nonjudgmental and supportive style provides a portal leading us to our gifts and unleashing a world where we can live as sovereign beings."

—**Marlina Oliviera, principal and founder of Richmond Academy, Canada**

"In this book, Bedrick wields lightning: his insights strike, and suddenly, in that moment, I see everything. I see why women keep dieting, keep failing, keep thwarting ourselves, keep ending up face down in a puddle of shame and misery. I see that no part of this cycle of failure reveals any defect in us. I see that in spite of the pressures of patriarchy to make ourselves small in every sense, we are mighty, all of us, that we can rise up from that puddle and engage with our bodies and our desires for food in a wholly different way, a way that teaches us what we yearn for in our lives, not just in our bellies.

I recognized pieces of myself in almost every woman's story. I raged at the voices that shamed them, so much like voices that have shamed me. I rejoiced in their realizations and in some ways even envied them. I want more of the "joy of no." I want to inhabit my full power. This is a book to read and re-read. This is a book that pokes at you at 3 a.m., whispering to you to turn around, cock your head, look from another angle. This is a book that helps you get free."
—**Ann Pierson D'Angelo, Litigation Support Manager, ACLU of Indiana, U.S.**

"After reading this book, you will see how weight is a symbolic messenger straight from our soul. Bedrick shares a tightly-woven dialogue between seventeen incredibly astute, wise, and powerful women who shared their intimate struggles with weight. In that exchange, we see how each woman unleashed their personal inner wisdom, and learn how much that wisdom has revolutionized their lives for the better in the years that follow."
—**Carolyn M. Riker, MA, LMHC, mental health counselor, U.S.**

"The self-development and healing fields are filled with aggressive messages of "Not good enough!" and "Need to manipulate, change, fix!" and Bedrick's approach feels like an oasis of nourishment in the middle of a vast and soul-destroying desert of shame. I'm grateful this book is encouraging a vital paradigm shift from one of domination to one of deep curiosity and reverence for life's mysterious wisdom.

When I met the women in this book, I fell in love with, and found myself in, every one of them and I felt deeply empowered while witnessing David Bedrick honoring the sacredness within each of their paths. His tender and respectful approach is pure alchemy, and there's deep soul medicine in reading as this magic unfolds."

—Samantha de Sienna, scholar at
Orphan Wisdom, England

"This book has that quality of triggering a reader's self-experiential healing process, like diving deep in the sea and collecting pearls below the dark surface. From the first page, I realized this book goes much further and wider than a book about issues with women's body and weight. It hits the deep core of our human existence: pain and suffering, being locked in a kind of protective but harmful cage and not being able to fully exist, enjoy, and satisfy our needs. It's additionally amazing that such a sensitive and compassionate book that goes deeply into all these issues is written by a man. Bedrick is an ally who contributes huge support and understanding to our female perspective."

—Zora Subotić, MS, clinical psychologist and
coauthor of *Stress, Trauma, Recovery*, Croatia

"I've balanced out bad drinking habits, avoided drugs, and I even quit smoking after 27 years of being a heavy smoker, but food has been the most difficult to balance. *You Can't Judge a Body by Its Cover* is guiding me deeper.

The questions Bedrick asks these women, I'm asking myself, and *whoo*! By getting to know the women in this book, I see how much women as a group are bombarded daily with different sorts of abuses we each experience individually. There's so much power in being shown how systemic and widespread this abuse is. It stops feeling personal. That alone is life-changing."

—**Lynn Richardson McDonald, U.S.**

"Bedrick shines a light on our society, which gaslights women's experiences and diminishes our power, forcing us into a little box. He teaches us to examine the desire behind our hunger so we can live the expression of our nature. I promise, you will find yourself in at least one of these stories, and likely more, and gain priceless insight into your own struggles surrounding body shame and disordered eating."

—**Stephanie Rosen, MD, pathologist, U.S.**

"These are stories of opportunities lost and regained, and a celebration of all the things we could be doing with our lives if we weren't busy wrestling with body shame. Whatever your gender, whatever your size, if you've ever equated your worth with your weight, you need to read this book."

—**Liz Scarfe, psychotherapist, Australia**

"David Bedrick's brilliance pierces through the veil of my own denial. In his uniquely gifted way of seeing the world, Bedrick lays out a case for the deep and surprising intelligence held in our bodies that doesn't cry out for changing or fixing, but rather, understanding, and integration. His work allows me to see, specifically that there are places within myself that I shame and marginalize on a regular basis despite decades of inner work. This book is truly a gift to all who struggle."

—Tanya Taylor Rubenstein, story coach, U.S.

"Who would have thought that within what is typically considered overeating could actually be the source of social change itself? This book is filled with so much love—it's so exciting, heartwarming, and relieving to hear people tapping into their true inner desires—that the hatred both from outside and within melts away."

—Katje Wagner, PhD, clinical psychologist, U.S.

"Bedrick's book moved me as both a woman and a psychologist. His point of view brings hope, empathy, and respect to women. Turns out it's the exact emotional cocktail required to kill the devastating shame associated with weight and body issues."

—Heidi Wells, PsyD, trauma and abuse specialist, U.S.

Praise for *Talking Back to Dr. Phil*...

"David Bedrick understands that real change or transformation requires challenging accepted dogma and then approaching problems with compassion and curiosity. A great advocate for stopping the madness of body hatred and dieting."

—Jane R. Hirschmann and Carol H. Munter,
authors, *Overcoming Overeating*,
and *When Women Stop Hating Their Bodies*

"At last someone is taking on Dr. Phil with good sense and great humor. Life isn't a sixty-minute show where people just come in for the laying on of hands. Life is about working it all out with family, community, and love. *Talking Back to Dr. Phil* is a must read."

—Nikki Giovanni, poet, seven-time NAACP Image
Award recipient and author of *A Good Cry*

Praise for *Revisioning Activism*...

"General readers will find comfort in these practical essays that offer hope to those who believe they must suffer silently and alone, while therapists will have their methodologies reaffirmed or challenged."

—Foreword Reviews, Winter 2017

YOU CAN'T JUDGE A BODY BY ITS COVER

DAVID BEDRICK, JD

17 Women's Stories of Hunger, Body Shame, and Redemption

BELLY SONG press

Santa Fe, New Mexico

Published by: Belly Song Press
518 Old Santa Fe Trail, Suite 1 #626, Santa Fe, NM 87505
www.bellysongpress.com

Managing editor: Lisa Blair
Cover design: Lisa Blair and David Moratto
Interior design and production: David Moratto

You Can't Judge a Body by Its Cover is factually accurate, except that names, locales, and minor aspects of some chapters have been altered to preserve coherence while protecting privacy.

Printed in the United States of America

ISBN: 978-0-9998094-8-8 (paperback) | 978-0-9998094-9-5 (kindle) | 978-1-7339011-4-7 (PDF) | 978-1-7339011-5-4 (ePub) | LCCN: 2020941326

LCSH: Body image in women--Case studies. | Weight loss--Psychological aspects--Case studies. | Women--Psychology--Case studies. | Shame--Case studies. | Physical-appearance- based bias--Case studies. | Discrimination against overweight persons--Case studies. | Self-actualization (Psychology) in women--Case studies. | Self-esteem in women--Case studies.

LCC: BF697.5.B63 B43 2020 | DDC: 306.4/613--dc23

For all you are, Lisa, my true companion

Contents

Foreword

⁓

I N A WORLD WHERE multitudes of "should" after "should" are
cast upon women because of body shape and weight, misogynistic inner and outer tyrannies exact a terrible toll. For over
thirty years, I've seen this firsthand while working in a residen-
tial program for women and children as they recovered from a
multitude of abuse issues. Perhaps this gives me an especially
keen ability to recognize David and this book as a rare and
paradigm-shifting gift to life's bruised people. I am amazed at
how he moves—with and despite the resistance. He befriends
and empowers the women in this book to engage their own
resistance. He encourages them to see what is right with them,
versus what they and others have said was wrong with them.

More than that, David unfolds before us the wrinkles and
creases that are overwhelmingly misidentified as flaws, hidden
within the warp and woof of our fabric. He skillfully steps
within the spaces, tears, and snags to catch hold of what is un-
raveling. He sees and hears, through his skills as a process work-
er, the places that are stronger than they appear at first sight.

With all his senses and instincts, he sits with these women as they piece together their challenges, slights, hurts, insights, and truths. With care and gentleness, he accompanies them methodically, tenderly, and skillfully into self-revelation.

When Vanessa, as a child, heard her father describe her as "husky," it set her on a path of feeling wrong in her body, and split her consciousness between looking at the world and imagining how the world was judgmentally looking at her. This web of disapproval kept her from pursuing her dreams. After working with David, she launched forward into stunningly heroic roles as an EMT, a firefighter, and another that provides advanced life support neonatal care in a birthing center. Imagine how much more impoverished the world would be if she hadn't worked with David to neutralize her limiting beliefs.

Jasmine came to the process wrestling with the complexities of body image as an African American woman, and the messages from this society that told her she wasn't worthy of shining. In spite of that oppressive lie, she came to embrace being seen. She came to relish the boldness of her colorfulness.

I was deeply moved when Kelly became the person who could state—no ifs, ands, or buts—exactly what she wanted. David journeyed with her as she confronted the condemning voice. When Alexis found her power to use the word *no*, she found her love of self inside that one voiced syllable. I felt like cheering! You will too.

Power, wisdom, inner courage, and intelligence emerge as David and the women share learning. He does not operate in the "power over" mode of so many therapeutic interactions. He is *with*. He runs with, sits with, and ventures into the winds of healing, in solidarity with each awesome woman. What others have chastised, shamed, dismissed, misinterpreted, and invalidated, he recognizes as wisdom, intelligence, and love seeking to be heard and witnessed.

David shows pure love and respect for these women, and we can see that his way of being, combined with his training and respect for each woman, is unconditional. Each woman in this book accepted the invitation, at a soul level, to reside within herself and to live well because of his demonstrated and sustained faith in their abilities to recognize their own answers.

I invite you to feel the peace, flow, and excitement of their stories as you read this book. Get comfortable. Hear and sense the rhythm and rhyme, the synchronicity of flow, as he embarks upon enabling and facilitating wellness. The magic of this book is that it's not only meant to show you what other women have transcended and re-embraced. Your gifts await you, too. After reading this book, you will never listen to and witness yourself and others the same way again.

—INDIA ELAINE GARNETT, M.DIV.

Preface

"You get to the general by focusing on the particular."

—Ta-Nehisi Coates

T HIS IS NOT a general theory of weight loss. I am not going to put before you the seven steps, phases, or foods that will help guide your diet strategy.

This is not another weight-loss guide. I will not bank on your body shame, your hope for greater esteem, or even your health.

This is a protest and an alternative to looking at our bodies through a lens that others created—eyes that look at our bodies without acknowledging the brutal forces of cultural bias that tear down the expression of women's intelligence, power, and beauty; eyes that don't consider our personal history, our inner demons, our clashes with the culture's searing judgment, or our deepest unmet hungers; eyes that are without compassion or deep understanding. Eyes that shame.

These eyes judge our bodies like a book by its cover—without the details, stories, and interiority of experience that brings the characters to life and moves our eyes to tears, our voices to cry out, our bodies to cringe. They judge, blind to the complexities and paradoxes, the heroism and the reasoning, the wisdom and the grit beyond the cover that awaken our hearts to the humanity of the characters and our own.

For example, if you search "weight loss," you will need to wade through pages of links before you read about a woman raped as a girl who feels safer in her big body; before you read about how people do their very best to address their deeper hungers by eating certain foods; before you learn that only five percent of women are successful at sustainably losing weight; before you learn that eighty-one percent of ten-year-old girls are dieting regardless of their BMI index; before you learn that ninety-seven percent of women have violent voices in their heads about their bodies; before you learn that being overweight, even mildly obese, is not a health risk while gaining and losing lots of weight *is* a risk; before you read about how a patriarchal culture that objectifies women's bodies and circumscribes the expression of their power is inextricably woven into weight loss efforts; before you learn that women derail their efforts to lose weight, in part, because they resist the self-hating and body-shaming attitudes that inform their initial motivation to lose weight; before you learn that the diet industry amasses over $70 billion, and it banks on women's body shame and perceived failure around weight.

In these pages, I offer you seventeen stories of individual women who open the door to their souls: stories of shame and self-love, victimization and empowerment, being small and being big, fear and hope. Stories that are both powerful and intimate. These are the stories from bodies impacted by sexism and racism, rape and harsh parental criticism, and by the deepest hungers for an authentic life.

You will notice that I never speak about how much the women in these stories weigh or how much weight they gained or lost. This is because this kind of measuring, summing oneself up by scales, or promising my readers that if they read my book they will lose weight, is one more snake oil offering. Despite the conventional and agreed on notion that weight ultimately comes down to an objective outer measurement, this is mostly untrue. Further, thinking that the issue of weight loss must be approached by the numbers overlooks the more powerful and meaningful ways body size and eating are expressions of who we really are on the inside.

The women in this book were not successful or unsuccessful. They began a process of self-understanding, of dropping the shame that bound them to a self-abusing lens about their bodies. They began a process of learning to express their power, creativity, beauty, and intelligence with themselves, in relationships, and in the world. They became more empowered leaders and social agents. They began embracing their sovereignty, defining themselves as an authority, and living a more authentic path as they unfold their life project in a bolder and more self-loving manner.

How did I, a relatively thin white man, come to write a book about the pain and shame that women suffer?

Multiple times each year between 2002 and 2009, I taught a class on critical thinking. The final project was to write a paper where students used the knowledge and skills to "think through" any issue they chose. Many women chose to write about weight loss and dieting.

Moved by the regularity of this topic, I asked some of the women why they had chosen the topic. My heart was touched; my mind grew both furious at the internalized sexism they revealed and passionate to understand a deeper and more insightful paradigm.

I responded to my sensitized heart and mind by seeking

volunteers to do a series of psychological interviews. Volunteers were offered my support and insight, as well as a chance to tell their story in a way that would be useful to others, in return for consenting to my recording the interviews and using what I had learned to educate others, including using the transcripts for future publication.

Twenty-one people volunteered. At the time I was surprised that it was only women. I am no longer surprised. While an urge for diversity was partially satisfied by having women of color participate, I wrestled with whether I should seek to find some men to participate. After some reflection, an inner voice calmed me: "Only women volunteered because that is what you are meant to learn about and write about."

This immediately rang true. I have always felt called, even ethically obligated, to bear witness to the stories and experiences of people who suffer under mainstream culture's marginalization. For the purposes of this book, that meant to bear witness to the stories and experiences of women at a critical location: the body.

As a psychologically minded person, I was moved to bear witness not only to peoples' outer stories but to their *inside* stories of internalization of oppressive regimes, of disavowed hungers and needs, of unvoiced sufferings and truths. In writing this book, I tasked myself with titrating the truth, suffering, beauty, and wisdom of these women's stories into a medicine capable of freeing bodies from shame and enlightening shaming minds, a medicine that would be both curative for the individual and the culture at large.

Toward that end, this book goes beyond outing and deconstructing the forces of sexism, misogyny, and shame. There are already great books in this area, including the brilliant work of

Hirschmann and Munter, *When Women Stop Hating their Bodies*, and the intimate self-love story in *Hunger* by Roxane Gay. Resisting the forces that breed self-blame and shame is a critical step, but it's not enough. The way we eat, what we eat, and the specific criticisms of our body's shapes are locations of particular and profound intimacy waiting to be awakened. In this way, this book takes another step: it redeems the body and its hungers by offering a vision of self-love that touches each detail, revealing not only a shame to be resisted but an intelligence about who these women are, what powers they bring to bear, and the nature of their gifts waiting to be lived.

Just to be clear, it is not that I think men's stories of body shame are not worthy to study and write about. They are. I hope someone, perhaps even I, will tell those stories.

It is my hope that as you read these stories, your eyes for yourself and for others will change. Instead of seeing through critical and judgmental eyes, it is my hope you will become curious and compassionate, self-trusting and self-protective, and aware of the brutal forces of cultural bias that tear down the expression of women's intelligence, power, and beauty. It is my hope that the revealed humanity of these women allows you to bear witness to your own.

The Acorn in the Fortress

WHAT IF YOUR hunger—that force that pulls you to the ice cream aisle, and guides your hands to take seconds when you swore you didn't even feel like having firsts—reviled, suffered, and deplored, resolution-foiling, *that hunger*, was the misunderstood sage of your body, rattling its cage inside the fortress of your soul?

What if your resistance to dieting, your sabotaging of your plan, your unwillingness to continue, yo-yoing, on and off again —what if that were a message of self-love, against self-hatred and shame?

What if your body size and shape also held intelligence, protecting you, taking up space, with power as far-seeing as your dreams?

What if your hunger were the teacher you've been waiting for?

What if your hunger would love to tell you the answers and is just waiting for you to listen?

Of the people who go on a diet, ninety to ninety-five percent either stay the same weight or gain weight, and you can bet most of those people feel like failures. But in fact, they're not lazy, stupid, or undisciplined. Failing at dieting masquerades as a problem of willpower and discipline, but it's just as potent and complex as any other psychological issue or physical illness.

My research has shown that resistance to dieting is a healthy response to the shaming that is baked into what drives people to try to lose weight. Because people naturally resist shame and self-hatred, they subconsciously undermine diets motivated by these feelings. At the very least, our diet resistance is a "screw you" to garden-variety external and internalized shaming, exacerbated by sexism, racism, classism, trauma, and abuse.

Our hunger sends us dispatches from who we really are—our deepest needs, wants, and desires—because even though we think we can ignore, silence, and push them aside, however submerged our authentic self is, it remains a powerhouse. We can channel these forces for our own good, or we can continue to be punished by punishing ourselves. I came to this understanding through my studies of a little-known branch of psychology called Process Work, and I want to share it with you.

The Genesis of Process Work

When I learned about Process Work, or Process-oriented Psychology, founded by Drs. Arny and Amy Mindell, it changed my life *and* my practice. Arny Mindell is an MIT physicist turned Jungian analyst. Process Work was originally called Dreambody Psychology, and once I describe it more, you'll see why.

According to Jungian psychology, dreams tell us things we don't know about ourselves. If a person is shy but has a dream in which they are being loud and extroverted, that tells us that the person may also have outgoing qualities that they've been unaware of—and when they do express them, they become more whole, more *themselves*.

Arny Mindell expanded this tenet to encompass the body and its physical symptoms. He developed gout as a young man, and became interested, wondering, "Why don't I understand what's happening with my body?" He went to a hospital in Zurich and worked with people who were terminally ill.

For example, he might ask, "Can you tell me about your physical illness?"

And a person might say, "Yes, I have a tumor."

"Can you describe the experience of the tumor?"

The patient might press the knuckle of one hand against the palm of the other, slowly grinding his knuckle against his hand. This was his way of expressing what was happening inside his body.

Then Mindell might ask him about his dreams.

"I had a dream about a car going down the road really fast and then smashing into a wall."

Mindell saw that they both carried the same information. One was expressed by a dream, and the other with the somatic experience of the knuckle against the palm. Body symptoms and nighttime dreams mirror each other.

The psyche dreams when we're asleep, and the body dreams in the form of illnesses, physical symptoms, even body movements or body language when we're awake.

That might give rise to the question, "Is everything psychosomatic; does the psyche cause the body to be ill?" No. But the body and psyche mirror each other. The body has the same information that the psyche has. It's as if the body is dreaming in the form of the manifestation of symptoms, manifesting, somatically, what we are unaware of. I see this as the Big Bang in psychology, an empirical answer to the mind-body question as it has developed over the last fifty years.

My own Big Bang was to apply this to weight issues. When someone wants to be small, thin, but their body is heavy and resists losing weight, that's an example of how the body is dreaming something different and expressing something meaningful that the person is often unaware of—a message that needs to be addressed, a message that may resist any and all weight-loss strategies.

Sizes, hungers, and shapes of bodies are expressing something meaningful. If we just support a person losing weight, with exercise and diet, we're trying to get rid of the weight and eating habits without addressing the meaning, integrating its intelligence. We're treating the body shape and size as the mainstream culture does, as almost all weight-loss programs do: as pathologies to get rid of.

I learned the same is true with our hungers. We can't get rid of them because they are expressions of who we are. We may think, "I shouldn't eat pizza," but the hunger for that pizza is a manifestation of who we are, a part of us that will also be expressed in our dreams.

The paradigm we're accustomed to is an allopathic one. What's wrong with me? I need to fix it, eliminate it:

"I have a fever of 102 degrees, and I need to get it back to 98.6."

"If I have heartburn, I need to get rid of the stomach acid."

It's based on the assumption that *the thing that is wrong with me is not me. I can get rid of it and become the pure me, the right me, the "healed" me.* But psychological difficulties are different. If we get angry but try to get rid of it, we only end up suppressing parts of ourselves. I can't get rid of myself; I must become my-self. I can't get rid of my hungers and body size; I must become them—not the size and eating habits themselves, but the intelligence expressed in my size and habits.

Thus, if we just tell a person to change their eating habits—if we try to get rid of the drive to eat and the energy behind it —we'll be in conflict with the person's deep nature, and we're not going to win. Less than five percent—some say eight or ten percent—of people are successful at losing weight and keeping it off. They're trying to get rid of something that's saying, "I'm hungry for something. You're not getting rid of me, I may be an expression of your deepest desires. Help me live them."

More specifically, if you love to eat ice cream, that hunger for the ice cream is part of you. It represents, is a stand in for, your hunger for something important in your life.

Or, if you are not happy with the roundness of your belly and want to get rid of it, I understand, of course, but there's a message your body is trying to tell you in the form of the round-ness. Unless you encounter, acknowledge, and integrate that message, you'll be frustrating your body's desire to be under-stood and keeping an issue unresolved. The body and the psyche are incredibly resistant to being denied, erased, or disavowed.

It doesn't mean you can't lose weight, but if you try to lose weight without addressing the intelligence in your current body and hungers, you will miss the message and likely be unsuccess-ful. And, perhaps worst of all, you will miss the biggest factor in making any deep and difficult change: you won't learn to love yourself and live a life that is truly yours.

As I worked with the women in this book, I saw that when we were able to identify and get to know these expressions, and ad-dress them, some women were successful at losing weight, but all were capable of changing their lives to be more fulfilling and self-loving, because they were becoming more themselves.

Process Work in Action

I knew I needed to learn more about Process Work once I heard about it, so I went to a workshop on the Oregon coast. Its focus was physical symptoms and working with the body's illnesses and disabilities.

There were over a hundred of us sitting in a circle. Arny Mindell asked if anyone wanted to volunteer to work with him. A woman raised her hand and said she wanted to work on her cerebral palsy. She went up to Arny.

He asked, "What's it like to have cerebral palsy?"

"I have a lot of difficulties. I can't control the muscles in my body so well, so when my mouth and tongue try to form words, it's not easy for other people to understand me. I can see that they are afraid to ask me to repeat myself, so they just nod. I want to be understood. Also, people think I'm mentally less able, which is not true. These things pain me. I also have a hard time walking. My stability isn't great."

We were all moved by her struggles and how people viewed her in ways that stung, hurt, or injured. An important healing occurs when a person is understood and shown compassion.

He then said, "So you've learned to try to adapt to the world we have, you've learned to speak more clearly. How did you learn to walk as well as you do?"

"A lot of physical therapy. I have to use my muscles very deliberately. For me, walking is like walking meditation just to move from point A to B."

He then asked something that blew my mind. "What would

happen if you didn't act like the person you're supposed to be, if you didn't try to walk in the way most people believe is normal?"

"I'm afraid I'd fall," she said.

"If you could hold on to my arm, would you let your body do what it wants to do in its own way?" It's as if he were saying, "Would you allow cerebral palsy to be something not to overcome, but something that moves your body in a way unique to you?" Tears ran down my face as I saw him not treat her like there was something wrong with her. He believed in her as she was.

She agreed to it. I watched as she began to move. She wasn't moving forward in a linear manner; she was moving in a circular way, her feet moving ever so slowly, one moving to the side, and the other then moving to meet it. He went with her as she held onto his forearm. Then she started to move faster and to look more stable than when she had walked up to join him, when she was trying to be "normal." He dropped his arm. She let go and the circles turned into a spinning motion, like a top, like a child would. Her spinning became faster and faster. I heard a sound come from her: "Whoooo! Whooo!" The joy, ecstasy, was infectious.

He shouted out, as she was spinning and "whooing," "What kind of person are you?"

"I'm a wild woman!" she responded.

More tears poured down my face. I saw that he believed in this thing that was called an illness. He just didn't see the diagnosis as the truth. She was doing something that expressed who she really was—and I saw the person underneath the behaviors that attempted to conform to expectations. She was seen for who she was and experienced herself that way, in her own eyes. Her cerebral palsy didn't go away, but I never saw a "healing" more beautiful.

That night, after the seminar, we had a dance party. Sandy was there spinning, the rest of us joined in her spinning as well. We wanted "what she was having"; we wanted to be more like her.

I spent ten days in that workshop, and then I left everything. I left the company I had just taken twelve years to build. I left the city, my lifestyle—and I left my partner—to go study with Arny Mindell. I wanted to believe in people the way he did. I wanted to not look at people as if they had something wrong with them. I thought, "That's how it's supposed to go. People are amazing the way they are. We just don't know how to look at each other." We've been hypnotized by the expectations of how we are supposed to look and be. It's a constant assault. It's literally a shame.

I recently saw a meme depicting a woman on a train. Where an ad would be, a message read, "In a society that profits from your self-doubt, liking yourself is a rebellious act."

The Shame Fortress

People often experience themselves through shame's lens. That lens imprisons the self, the soul, keeping us from the truth of our own experiences. I call this the shame fortress. Let me explain.

Shame has many meanings. Most people define shame as a painful feeling. But in my view, shame is a dynamic that starts with an assault. Assaults hurt, they injure and cause reactions—anger, withdrawal. Shame enters the scene when the assault, hurt, injury, or reactions are dismissed ("That wasn't such a big deal, why are you so sensitive?"), denied ("You're lying, making it up, that didn't really happen"), or gaslighted ("Your reactions are because something is weird or pathologically wrong with you, not because of the assault"). These leave people feeling, believing, and internalizing shame's message: "I am feeling, sensing, reacting the way I do because something is wrong with me."

"Something is wrong with me;" that's the sine qua non of shame.

For example, let's say that a child is assaulted by a parent. The other parent looks away, or dismisses, minimizes, or simply doesn't see it. What happens psychologically? The assault needs to be addressed in the short term, whether it is physical, psychological, or both. The "cut" needs a bandage. However, the way the other parent witnesses the event has a longer-term impact. The child is hurt by the assault, but the child internalizes the witnessing parent's viewpoint. So, when this child becomes an adult, they may never seek help, never talk about being abused, or make any effort to heal their injury for one simple reason: they have internalized the viewpoint of the parent who witnessed the event and now they too dismiss, minimize, or deny its occurrence.

While the initial assault, like any wound, requires addressing and redressing, the insufficient witnessing wraps the wound in shame, like a bandage that is now bacteria-laden, infecting the person's beliefs, convincing them that their pain and suffering is a result of their own inadequacy.

As the child grows older, they may experience a myriad of difficult feelings and patterns of behavior: fear, insecurity, self-hatred, boundary confusion, cyclic patterns of difficult relationships, substance abuse, or over- and under-eating, but they may never get to the root of the problem. They may never make a genuine and loving inquiry into the reasons for their suffering. Instead, they ask "What's wrong with me?" and conclude that the feelings and patterns of behavior they suffer from exist because something is wrong with them, not because something happened to them. They conclude that their symptoms should be treated as pathologies to be gotten rid of, instead of intelligent signs of our story, our experience, our natural intelligence. This is the essence of shame.

In summary, the shamed person turns away from their own experience, truth, intuition, hesitancies, reactions, and feelings. Their needed defenses and boundaries are dismantled; their true self is disbelieved, not trusted, and not nourished as it becomes more and more hidden from themselves and others around them.

When people come to therapy citing the assaults, abuses, and traumas they experienced, progress is imminent. When people come to therapy citing all the reasons why there is something wrong with them, progress becomes ever more difficult.

A fortress is formed inside the person—a place that's unreachable to the self, where parts of the person that have been shamed are locked up. And also inaccessible: they're unable to see what's going on, to identify why they are moved to act and feel the way they do. This vault of blankness prevents them from embracing the intelligence of their impulses.

What's locked up in the shame fortress has so much potential for a person's growth. It's like an acorn inside the fortress, an acorn that never sees the sun, but if it were let loose, it could become a majestic oak tree.

The Acorn in the Body

When it comes to our dieting culture, assaults are ever present. They might be someone calling you fat when you have more than a slight build, or the persistent messages about what is and is not beautiful, healthy, or responsible. For example, the iconic cereal commercial that asked, "Can you pinch an inch?" Or the

BMI charts that offer debunked and outdated weight ranges, the schoolyard bully, insidious norms for young girls. Injuries abound.

But these assaults are almost never witnessed. First of all, the hurt and harm are not expressed in words, tears, or screams. If we can't hear or see the pain, how can they be witnessed? Second, the assaultive messages are not confronted. A non-shaming witness has a reaction to assaults; we naturally resist, confront, or protect the injured. However, in our culture, assaults come in the form of jokes and accepted critiques. Third, the ramifications of the violence, be it self-hate, depressions, and anxieties, or torn-down esteem and addictions, are not seen as manifestations of the assault on women's bodies. Instead, women are pathologized. Their depressions and anxieties are thought to arise from their faulty psychology as opposed to outer oppression. Even when the ramifications are obvious direct results of a culture of body shaming, such as women hating their bodies, feeding or starving their bodies, and having their esteem tied to their body size and shape, women internalize the view that they suffer from a lack of self-discipline or some other psychological pathology.

Women not only internalize the assaults, the criticism, but also the viewpoint that all the pain they are experiencing is because something is wrong with them. When you ask me about my eating, I'm going to filter my answers through this viewpoint, which looks at myself not as a person who's intelligent, seeking meaning in my life, having a desire behind a desire, and being harmed. I'm looking at myself and seeing something that I not only hate but believe is screwed up. I am not a person in pain, a person with power, a person who can trust themselves. Instead, I am a person whose inadequacies, failures, and faultiness are causing health problems, and causing me to be unattractive.

xlii   David Bedrick, JD

We all collude in a blindness to the perpetration of assault on women's bodies. Together, we create a culture of shame.

This viewpoint comes from American culture: "It's easy to lose weight, just exercise and stop eating. Everybody knows that it's totally within your control." It's not totally within people's control, but we'll get to that. The dominant narrative is, "You're in this situation because you don't have discipline, you don't have willpower. There are things inside you that you haven't resolved, and you're self-medicating with food."

What's implied: "Something's wrong with me. If we cured my illness, all of a sudden I would be healthy, I'd have the perfect body, I would eat the right foods, get into a good relationship, find success, and have all the things I want. My life is not happening because I'm a screwed-up person. Fix me!"

If I approached that person, like many people would—a coach, a therapist, or a diet-program leader—and said, "Oh, great. Let me help you do that. I have lots of ways to help you lose weight," I'd have made a fundamental error, and that is I'm believing that losing weight is motivated only by reasons of self-care and health and not body shame and self-hatred. Worse, I become allied with their shame and self-hatred, however unintentional. It's as if I'm saying, "I agree with your assessment. Of course you hate yourself; of course something is wrong with you. Your eating habits and body size are not indicators of anything meaningful. There is no story to be told. There is no pain to be addressed. There is no assault you are responding to. There is no hunger you have for life behind your hunger for food. The answer is simple, 'You need to lose weight.'"

Because, isn't it? Let's say the person is 350 pounds. Wouldn't it be good to lose weight if they have a heart condition? Yet if the motivation, however logically positive, is coming from a place of unexamined shame, they will very rarely succeed. And they may become more blind to the meaning and intelligence behind their eating patterns and weight gain. For example, if that woman gained weight after an earlier sexual assault and her large body left her feeling safer, then going along with her weight-loss agenda is tantamount to dismissing her need for safety. It may even deepen the pain and trauma of her abuse because I am acting as if there is no good reason to be 350 pounds. In a way, I am denying her abuse. If she feels unsafe in the world, for good reason, how successful do you think her diet plan will be when losing weight makes her feel less and less safe in the world?

For instance, I might say, "Why do you want to lose weight?"

"Well, I'd be much healthier if I could lose two hundred pounds."

"Really? Tell me about that."

"I really don't look good. My clothes look bad on me and I hate shopping for new ones, because they look even worse. People think I don't have any control over myself. I can't walk up a hill. Who's going to want to be with somebody who looks like this?"

When the diet program is allied with shame and self-hatred, very few people can motivate themselves positively for long. Most people can't stand *not* liking themselves. The first thing a person's psyche wants to do, in a reflexively healthy act, is stop: "I don't want to continue hating myself!"

How do they self-correct? "Eat the darn pizza again, walk away from a weight-loss program inextricable from self-hatred and shame, and let myself have everything I want."

Conventional diet programs punish the healthy part of a person, because the healthy part is saying, "I need to love myself. I don't want to criticize myself incessantly. I want to take care of the deep needs that I have, even when those needs are hidden in disturbing eating habits. I can't stand thinking that I am somehow defective." Influencing people to feel bad about a good part of themselves is crazy-making and results in resuming old habits.

You can lose weight while being motivated by self-love. But to do that, you have to know what you're doing with food. What desire are you trying to satisfy behind the desire for nachos, or ice cream, or pie?

You can't love the parts of yourself you're not yet aware of. These parts of you are waiting for you to notice them and let their wisdom launch you forward. These parts need a loving not a shaming witness.

What Don't You Like about Your Body?

There are so many judgments about the way bodies should look, act, and feel. These are externally imposed viewpoints that become internalized because they are so pervasive. These imposed viewpoints come from sexist and cultural biases and lead to eating disorders, shame, self-hatred, and psychological anguish.

A major study showed that being overweight or mildly obese does not pose health risks, unless the person is eating health-harming food. However, research does show that gaining and losing weight—yo-yo dieting (the most common result of any diet effort)—is more of a health risk. But if a person is eating healthfully, the weight itself is not a health issue.

Eating disorders, however, are a major health risk. They are often deadly obsessions with the body's shape and size. In fact, many women literally "see" their bodies as bigger than they are, even when looking at a photo or in the mirror. The stakes are that high; the myth needs to be exposed for what it is.

These hurtful cultural views assault people with their declarations of what it looks like to be normal, healthy, and attractive. Thus women come to believe that their bodies should be shaped differently. But the body says, "I'm not doing that. I'm not going along with that externally imposed belief." Just as the eating habits I spoke about above, the existing shape of the body has its own wisdom. Loving the body almost always means that we first learn about it.

So I ask my clients, "How do you not fit? What do you not like about your body?"

One of them said, "I don't like my belly, it pushes out. I don't like how big it is, how much room it takes up."

The body is saying, "I'm not so small. I'm bigger." The person is thinking, "I want to be smaller," but the body is not going along with that cultural and personal agenda. The body is a rebel.

I say, "Tell me about this big body. I want to get to know you. Tell me what bigness is like."

"My body is this big round thing in front of me. It's a bad thing. I'm worried that my boss will think I'm a slob, lazy, disorganized about taking care of myself and also other things."

I bring it into a somatic expression. I ask her to show me, with her arms and hands, what the big body in front of her is like. She brings them out in a kind of round ring, hands together. I ask her if I can press against those hands, and she agrees.

I feel her push back against my hands. It's a manifestation of what she is—she is pushing back.

"How come you resist my pushing?" I ask.

"I'm tired of shrinking. Making myself smaller. Having no boundaries. I refuse to play small any longer."

Her body's size and how it pushes out in front of her stands for that message and dreams of that boundary. It's wise. It's an expression of her authenticity and power. But her mind thinks it's bad, and she wants help getting rid of it. If someone says, "Sure, I'll help you get rid of it," they're trying to make her healthier, but also, her psyche hears, "Return to your socialized self. Listen to others, put away your opinions, be more agreeable and open," and the psyche responds, "I'm not doing that. Not again." Her weight-loss intention appears as a healthy one, but to the psyche it runs counter to her truth, her development. It denies and dismisses who she really is, treating it as a psychological problem to get over, rather than a valid and fundamental urge to authenticity and selfhood. In short, it shames her. However, the natural impulse to fill herself out, to take up the space that is rightfully hers, is powerful, so powerful that all the body shame and self-hatred cannot lead to weight loss. Any strategy for this woman must address this underlying urge in relationships and the world in addition to conventional disciplines regarding food and exercise.

Cravings as Body Expressions, or the Secret in the Sauce

When people are ashamed of their bodies, they are often also ashamed about their eating habits. It's important to look at these habits. If it's ice cream, I want to find out what the client is experiencing when she's eating ice cream, because there's something meaningful embedded in that craving. I want to know what she is *deeply* craving. A person will often think, "I eat too much of this to comfort myself." Sometimes that's true, but it's almost always more nuanced than that. I see it more as, "I'm hungry for something. I'm lacking something. I want something. I'm not getting enough of something. I want a different kind of life or way of living."

People feel a deep hunger for *something* but conflate that feeling with being hungry for a particular food. Why? Because reaching for what they are actually hungry for has been forbidden or rendered risky in a culture or family. Living their hungers literally outs them as individuals who are unwilling to be controlled by norms and accommodations. The food never satisfies their deeper hunger, so they often keep eating it, teased by the possibility of deeper fulfillment, unaware of what their soul is actually craving.

I ask people about their favorite foods to help them discover this desire behind the desire, the hunger behind the hunger. If I'm going to help a person who voices a weight-loss agenda, then I want to help them make a life change that allows them to get to know what they are more deeply hungry for, and find ways to satiate those specific hungers in ways that are closer, more true to the essence of that hunger and don't lead to remorse and self-shaming.

Our deeper body intelligence chooses the food and the tastes we aren't getting enough of. People are constantly looking for flavors to infuse into their lives, like when they decide which movie to watch (scary, romantic, meditative, funny), or vacation to go on (adventurous, beachy, opulent, artsy), but they're usually not conscious of their desire when they're doing that with food.

To access a person's specific hungers, I have to ask the person in a way that brings out this deep intelligence. The intelligence cannot be found in their ideas or opinions; it can only be found in their actual experience. Ideas and opinions are often disconnected from the body experience and are almost always fused with simplistic cultural ideas that invariably carry criticism, condescension, and shame along with them. Here's an example:

I once worked with a woman who really liked a certain kind of ice cream.

I asked, "What kind?" because I wanted to know what she was tasting. Otherwise, her mind and her ideas about herself were going to give me an answer along the lines of "Well, I don't know, because I'm a pig." That's a really harsh thing to say; that's the shamed mind speaking. But all too often people say things like that about themselves (as you'll see in Kimberly's chapter). Not only is that criticism harsh and shaming, it is entirely absent of any actual experience of eating the particular food. That's what shame does—disconnects us from our experience, from ourselves.

"Salted caramel ice cream."

"Imagine having a spoonful of it. Imagine putting it in your mouth. Close your eyes. Put the salted caramel ice cream in your mouth and tell me what happens. Make a sound."

I said those things because I wanted to know what she was tasting *for*. Her tongue was smart, her mouth was smart. She was looking for a flavor, just like we look for flavors in relationships —like a spicy relationship, a sweet relationship, a soothing relationship, a zingy relationship.

If a person is craving spicy chips, it might be because they want more spice in their relationship, but they don't grab their partner and say, "I want more intimacy, more spice." That could be awkward and might lead to rejection. The psyche whispers, beneath the level of awareness, "This spicy dish tastes a little bit like what I'm searching for." If you tell that person, "No more spicy chips," you're taking it away without helping them to get more spice into their lives. It's not going to work out well.

"How does the ice cream taste?"

She answered, "Mm-hmm. I hear the angels singing."

"That's so beautiful. Tell me about angels singing."

"Well, in the morning, I go for a walk and I pass by the church. And sometimes there's a choral group singing, and they sound like angels."

"Say more to me about your spiritual life," I said, responding to what she had shared: the sensation of eating ice cream reminds her of something spiritual.

"Well, I pray very hard."

I could see her body language change from communicating enjoyment to a stiff posture. Some people, when they think about practicing their religion, take on a rigid and punitive energy.

"David, I'm trying to be a good mother, and I'm trying to be a good wife, and I'm trying to be a good religious person."

"Yes, that's a kind of spiritual view: 'I'm going to be a good person.'" Yet that doesn't sound glorious or angelic—or fun. Her spirituality needed more singing, more glory. That's a whole different flavor of spirituality. She needed to listen to more gospel music and spend less time sitting rigidly, trying to will herself into being a good person. The wisdom within her ice cream–eating practice was that she was reaching out for her heavenly reward on earth, instead of limiting herself to grim piety. Her soul knew she should experience joy in her spirituality, and so when she ate the ice cream, she was tasting that.

One of the stories in this book focuses on Erica, who felt bad about habitually consuming caramel mochas at Starbucks. She thought she would be thinner if she could stop drinking them. She also felt bad about the expense and time involved.

"I have to drive twenty minutes to get one, and it takes time away from being home with my husband. But I still want it."

The conventional approach to this situation would be, "Just stop doing it! Think of the consequences." But it's not useful or effective. You'll read the whole story in chapter five, but we did a somatic exercise that revealed that her psyche was interpreting the coffee drink as happiness. Her diet plan included finding more ways to experience happiness, outside of that steaming, creamy cup of chocolaty sweetness. If I had only told her to quit drinking caramel mochas, her need for happiness would be unaddressed, and she'd go back to unconsciously sourcing her happiness at Starbucks, because otherwise, her life would seem unremittingly bleak.

Is everyone looking for angel choirs in their mouthfuls of tasty food? No, somebody else is going to taste something totally different, and they're going to look for a different kind of flavor. Even if another client also really loves ice cream, they might say, "I like chocolate with chocolate chips and fudge on top."

"Why?"

"I like the chocolate, on top of chocolate, on top of chocolate, because I want indulgence."

The indulgence that person's looking for is pointing to a need to feel indulgence in other areas of her life, particularly in a life where indulgence itself is looked down on, seen as immoral, undisciplined—shame-worthy.

And yet until now, when people seek help to lose weight, they rarely get beyond the surface. zA nutritionist might say, after instructing a client to write down everything they eat and reviewing the list, "Aha, I see that you eat a lot of pizza. Here's what you should do about that. Let yourself have pizza once a week, but it should be the frozen diet version, or eat one with a whole wheat crust, without cheese." They don't ask, "What kind of pizza is your favorite? Do you like sausage on it, or a thick crust, or a crispy crust? Do you like sausage or pepperoni? Do you like the cheese melting and dripping off the side? Or do you just like little dots of cheese?"

I want to help them come in contact with their actual experiences. If you just say, "Stop eating pizza," then they are still hungry for both the easy fix, pizza, and that undiscovered thing behind it.

"I love this smoky brick oven pizza, with duck."

"What do you like about that?"

"There's an interesting contrast with the cheese, that smokiness. It's salty, creamy, smoky, acidic from the tomatoes."

Now I'm in, connecting with the desire behind the desire. Dear reader, can you taste the fullness of strong flavor, like a "pow" of flavor?

"What do you really want?"

"I want to go on a date with a man."

"What kind of man?" I'm staying with the specific, not broadening it out to a generic search for love and connection. "A heavy one? A bearded one? A clean-shaven one? Which guy really connects to that flavor? The relationship needs some 'pow.' Tell me about life, your relationship with all those flavors. What would your workplace look like with that pow? What are the flavorless, monotone, neutral parts of your life? Are you hanging around with all the same kind of people all the time and getting bored? Maybe you need some diversity in your life."

You cannot replace your hunger with just anything; it must be something that has the right taste, what you're really hungry for.

I'm not interested in taking foods away from you so you can

lii   David Bedrick, JD

merely change your body shape and size (because, among other reasons, that seldom works). I'm interested in the desire behind your desire, which holds an intelligence that can lead you to the life you want. Not so you can just lose weight, but so you can attain your best possible life, so you can live the expression of your nature, your authentic self.

Physical Expressions, or the Secrets in the Soma

When I ask people questions about their eating, the first thing they express is their ideas and opinions about themselves, and most of them are negative. People's sense of themselves and their bodies and what they eat is often wrapped up in shame. Shame answers the question.

"I'm lazy and I'm no good. I'm comforting myself and I have to get over that."

I want a way to get past that viewpoint, which is simply a shaming viewpoint: "I'm a lousy no-good piece of dung." And sometimes it's more sympathetic: "I'm a lousy piece of dung because I got hurt as a child. But I'm still a lousy piece of dung, okay?"

What I hear is, "There's nothing interesting, worthy of love, intelligent, alive, natural, or gifted inside of me. I'm just this thing." That's how it looks through shame's eyes. Shame not only objectifies the person but blocks the path to any real self-knowledge or self-love.

How do we get access to the information on the other side of that strong viewpoint? It answers all questions with the same answer: "I'm a no-good human being." "This is what's wrong with me." This is where many "diet professionals" think, "Great, then buy my product." A person who feels bad about themselves is an easy person to market to: "I feel really, really terrible about myself, and you're giving me a hope that I can experience a transformation, especially one where I feel better about myself. If I have the money, I'm going to pay."

One way of getting to know the self, the soul or the spirit of the person, is to ask them body questions. The body doesn't lie. And how do you ask the body questions? You have to talk to the body in its own language.

When a person is talking about how something feels in their body, oftentimes they'll start moving and they don't even know they're doing a little associated dance. The body wants to communicate so badly. When I ask people to talk about their favorite foods, inevitably they're dying to tell someone. The body is dying to *show* someone.

One of my clients really loved Guinness beer.

"What's it *feel* like when you have that Guinness beer?"

"It's chocolaty and dark and malty."

"Mmm, close your eyes and feel it in your body."

"It's a really good beer, it comes from Ireland."

Notice how her mind tried to take over.

"Those are good details, but in your body, when you have that rich and chocolaty beer, what does it feel like?"

I watch her sit back, sink into the chair. Her shoulders drop.

"Yeah, sit back, you're sitting back, stronger, in your chair."

"I feel a weightiness, sitting back in a leather chair, drinking my Guinness."

Maybe she needs that weightiness, or the feeling of being in a big chair: entitlement. The body knows it, but the mind doesn't always.

Or maybe she likes to order Guinness because bartenders

liv   David Bedrick, JD

can't just slosh it into the glass. They have to pour a bit, and then it needs to settle, and then pour some more, and wait. There's a wonderful contrast between the dark beer at the bottom and the amazing creamy foam at the top. Maybe she loves Guinness because it forces her to slow down, care for what she takes in, and savor it.

If my client said those things, I'd ask, "What's it like to have to slow down, to have something made for you, composed for you? Feel it in your body."

"I feel like I have to work all the time, my body's weary, my muscles are always ready to spring into action, my neck is tight. There's not enough of anything."

So after work, guess what? It's Guinness time.

"Four Guinnesses is a little bit much, five is really a lot, six, well, I shouldn't do that." The person who is drinking six Guinnesses criticizes herself, gets stuck in shame, and it becomes a vicious cycle, without realizing that her resistance to slowing down and savoring life is so great that it takes six Guinnesses to overcome it (at least for this moment).

What part of you wants the spice of being the life of the party, wants the angels singing in the ice cream, the slowing down of the Guinness? You have to love that part of yourself too, because if you love everything but that, you aren't loving the best of yourself, which is your own intelligence signaling the deeply needed experiences you aren't yet getting in your life.

A guy once came to me because he felt he was smoking too much marijuana. He and his friends liked to go out a lot and hear live music, and at some point during the night they'd go outside and smoke.

I ask him, "What's it like to smoke marijuana?"

"It's good, but I shouldn't do it."

He's coming from a shamed place, but I am hoping I can explore this topic more on a somatic level. I give him a little pen. "Here's my pen. Imagine this is marijuana." When he takes it, his body comes alive, while before, during his self-shaming comment, he had been slumped.

He puts the pen in his mouth, and his eyes light up like a beam.

"I see your face, it's lighting up. What's happening?"

He says, "I'm seeing the glow of the match, and my friends around me, in the dark, at night. We light this match, and I see their faces. Those are the deepest friendships I have." His eyes fill with tears.

He thinks he wants an experience of marijuana, but his body is saying, "The experience I want is the glow of the people I love around me." It's that match-strike moment he's looking for, more than actually smoking. That's very intimate for him. That's what he's hungry for.

When I notice what's going on in clients' bodies while they're talking about what they love to eat, or drink, or smoke, I can then pursue the nonverbal messages.

Engaging with Shame

I've talked about favorite foods, the messages of body movements, and shame, and you've seen how I assess what's motivating the person to want to go on a diet, change their body, or begin exercise. I have to be on the lookout for inner criticism and shame: notions, opinions, ideas about themselves that make them believe they're no good.

I have to identify these things, because they are rarely fully conscious, and I don't want them to continue to plague the person. We can't address what we can't yet see. When I ask, "Why do you want to lose weight? How do you feel about yourself when you look in the mirror? What happens when you put on your clothes in the morning?" I'm looking to find out if clients are looking at themselves, trying to motivate themselves, via shame and self-hatred. Self-hatred says, "You are ugly, undisciplined, disgusting." Shame says, "You deserve the criticism, the self-hate. You should be punished. You should feel bad. There is no other reason to have your body and eat the way you do other than the fact that you are insufficient, that something is wrong with you, that you need to be fixed." That viewpoint constitutes an internalized shaming witness. I want to help them find enough power to resist, fight, stand against that particular view.

I don't tell my clients, "Lose weight and then you'll love yourself." I say, "Love yourself, and then maybe you'll find yourself in a weight-loss plan that makes sense. Living your hungers and the intelligence of your body *is* loving yourself. If I'm going to help you love yourself, you have to address the self-hatred inside."

Respect, Relating, and Radical Belief

Part of engaging with my client's shame is working with them to dismantle their shame fortress: a psychological structure in which their deeper experiences and truths are hidden. How? I look at them through loving eyes. The lack of judgment weakens and dissolves shame. I am a non-shaming witness *for* them. When my clients experience this, they can begin to learn how to be that for themselves.

There are three aspects to this: *respect, relating,* and *radical belief.*

Respect

When I use the word *respect*, I'm not using the conventional definition. I think of the syllables: *spect*, spectate: to look at, and *re*spect: to re-look.

So, if a person says to me, "I don't like my body," I say, "What about it?" This attention is a form of looking. "Well, see this flesh here? I would like it to be firm, muscular. I don't want it to be *like this*."

"What's it like when it's *like this*?" I am re-looking.

"It's hanging."

Respect means I'm looking at that detail again. I want to look closely at that person. That way, I'm likely to find out that "hanging," "hanging out," "being looser," is going to be really helpful for them. Their eyes are seeing something they're against in themselves—not just flab, but looseness. If they're an uptight, type A overachiever, that person *needs* a lot of looseness, even though they're not yet identified with needing it. I look, and look again, so I don't miss that insight. Then, the person notices I'm interested in who they really are at a deeper level, I'm interested in what lies behind the disparagement. Respecting a person delivers the message, "I want to really see you, get to know you. I want to get beyond opinions and ideas about you; I want to get to know you." This attitude counters shame's barrier to self-knowledge and self-love.

Relating

When I talk about *relating*, I'm wondering, in this case, how she relates to her body's looseness if she thinks it's a weakness. If she relates to it as a problem, did she grow up in a certain way, thinking she always had to be on top? Does she have any compassion for how painful it is to look at her body in a certain way or to have a mainstream culture see her in a hurtful way? And can she relate to that part of herself in a different way? I relate to my client in this situation by spending time with her, while embodying this quality of looseness that she needs. I may wince or show expressions of empathy when she puts herself down. I might say, "Let's hang out together, instead of working on this diet program. Let's just chat with each other. Let's gossip about people who are thin and heavy." I'm relating to the person, while modeling and offering the quality she's looking for. And relating tends to neutralize shame, because then people feel *related to* as if they're a real person, not a bunch of problems, not a pathology in need of a cure, not an object, but a subject. Being related to in this way delivers the message, "You matter. How you think, how you feel, how you live matters." It delivers the message, "You are worthy of care, protection, and compassion."

Radical Belief
This last term means *I believe you* and I believe in you. You're going to tell me stories—about when you were young and how your father said you were chubby and put you down and beat you—and I'm going to listen to your stories and believe you. I'm going to believe that it hurts. And I'm going to believe in you, that this intelligence in you is guiding you to eat ice cream for a wise reason, and I can find out what the reason is, bring it from your unconscious into your conscious mind, where you can use it to make decisions about how to integrate the fulfillment of that deeper desire into your daily life.

Radical belief is the opposite of judgment, skepticism, and invalidating dismissal. People are so profoundly intelligent in so many ways, whether it's what we want to taste (and what that means), or the shape of our bodies.

When a client learns that she's doing something that makes sense (something she'd previously thought was a mark of failure), it's so freeing.

"I shouldn't be scared all the time. If I weren't, I'd be a courageous person."

"Tell me about being scared. Tell me a story about when you were scared."

Then she shares a situation in which it makes perfect sense to be scared.

"What a perfectly appropriate situation to be afraid of. How smart you were to notice that and look for ways to become safe again."

"You mean I'm not scared because I'm a broken, ineffective person who has to overcome their fear?"

"No, it was an intelligent response."

"Hmm. So my fear was intelligent. Maybe I can learn how to use it better."

Radical belief counters the essence of shame, that something is wrong with you, by offering a counter-attitude: something is absolutely right about you. When I affirm the deep being, rather than shaming the deep being, people come alive.

Shame is endemic in our culture, and tragically counterproductive. But when we put together those shame-dismantling qualities—respect, relating, and radical belief—people form a different viewpoint of themselves, a loving viewpoint, and it becomes a lot easier to make changes or to confidently decide, "This is not the change I want to make."

Role-playing

The intention of my work is to find out what's happening inside a person, instead of what their opinions are about their bodies. Our opinions about our bodies can be rather unfriendly, based on learned, internalized, negative reactions to ourselves. If I ask, "Why do you want to diet?" I'll often hear, "I'm unhealthy. I eat for all the wrong reasons." That's an opinion.

If a client shares the way she talks to herself, she might say, "I can't stand the way I am. Why can't I get through to you? I want to lose weight." I can then model how to respond by saying, "I don't like the way you talk to me." I'm reflecting an inner experience. That differs from a doctor's office conversation about weight that often shames. There is an inner dialogue going on, but most people aren't aware of it, or aware of it in a way that's constructive. I need to communicate with the part of a person that's in opposition to dieting, who says "Fuck you" to dieting, who seemingly derails all weight-loss efforts. If I don't find out who that is and what they truly want, any weight-loss strategy will fail when it meets that immovable, opposing force.

I once worked with a woman who complained that as soon as she began a diet, she'd start craving chocolate.

"And I don't even like chocolate!" That sounds crazy, but *crazy* to me means we're in a good place. People are not as logical, on a surface level, as they like to think they are. But our psychology has a deeper logic.

By using role-playing, I get to ask, "What's so good about eating chocolate?" I know that in the fight between losing weight and eating chocolate, the chocolate will win every time.

"Why eat chocolate? Because screw this diet shit, I don't want to diet. No, I won't drink more water and eat more salads.

I'll eat something I don't like because I enjoy saying no." There's a power in saying no; I give you the middle finger and it makes me light up like a Christmas tree. It's the beginning of life. There's no person, no agency, without saying no. This person's saying, "Learning and practicing to say no is exactly what I need to learn right now." Not being able to say no is worse than being heavy.

Saying no can be tough, especially for women, who are socialized to put others first, to be people-pleasers. Her weight-loss program will have to involve saying no in other areas of her life. She has to have a more empowered no, that's what her psychology is telling me. Her eating behavior says, "Help me say no." It's so gendered—to accommodate others. There's a history and a river of that conditioning. She's up against her inner struggle, but also against the flow of patriarchal violence that by its very nature violates her empowerment. It's embedded in religious paradigms. "Don't talk back." "Don't disrespect men."

What's a safe space to feel powerful? The space in which you go have some chocolate. By role-playing with a client, I can find out what the deeper need is and assist them in finding non-eating-related ways to meet those needs. Inevitably, the need, when expressed more directly, is a step in their needed growth and evolution as a soul.

Double Consciousness

In W.E.B. Du Bois's 1903 book, *The Souls of Black Folk*, he shares the concept of having more than one social identity—a splitting caused by the internalization of racism. Persons of color may see themselves as any individual does, but also sees themselves with a second pair of eyes, an oppressive viewpoint that judges them through the lens of often unconscious racist assumptions.

This concept is useful for other groups of people too. A woman might see herself with the internalized eyes of a culture that expects women to be slim and delicate. When she sees herself with those eyes, scanning from head to toe, those eyes hold a bias against the nature of her beauty, her power, her intelligence. But she may not even realize she's not looking at herself with her own eyes. She takes her critical opinion, her attitude of disgust, as the truth. This is the essence of internalized oppression, internalized sexism.

If one man in a group of women said, "I'm going to be the voice of the culture. You're fat. And you over there, you have saggy arms. And you in the blue shirt, your lips aren't full enough. And you, be quiet and listen to the men." Some women would wither, some would want to punch him out. Women would feel hurt, and many would tell him off.

But that voice is going on, all the time, inside women's minds, without a witness to resist it. When I role-play, I get to be that witness.

It's not just an aesthetic viewpoint, it's an attitude of disgust and a patriarchal viewpoint about women's sovereignty. The energy is very powerful. Instead of corroborating it, a non-shamed person would have the healthy response of hiding, running, finding allies, or punching back—not sitting in the vision of being put down and seen as disgusting. When I role-play, I out that disgusted viewpoint, interrogate it, make it conscious, and help to strengthen and often redirect the resistance to it.

Diet programs share that same internalized view and are complicit in the culture's views, capitalizing on women's internalized oppression and disgust in themselves rather than countering it. However unintended, they offer diets as a way to rid oneself of being down and disgusted. But it doesn't work, because most people have a secret superpower—a healthy level of defensiveness and resistance to these forces.

In short, diet programs feed on women's internalized sexism. One study measured the frequency of certain phrases women used when they talked to each other. One was "I don't know." A woman would say, "This is what I think..." and then after that conclude with "I don't know." The strong opinion would be paired with an invitation not to take them seriously. Why would an intelligent, otherwise clear person say that? The initial energy is strong, but the "I don't know" eases the appearance of strength —internalized sexism at work. The strength goes underground and is expressed sideways via body shape and size, and resistance to dieting. It's a delayed, indirect "Screw you."

Why is this important? When we talk about body shape and shame, eating and dieting are important because so many exercise their psychological power, shame, and self-hatred in that area. Food is a great place to dance those dances about power and resistance.

It's not just an individual issue; it's a cultural issue. For example, if I were the patient and you were my healer, you'd ask, "Where does it hurt?" I might say, "I get stomachaches," or "I have a frozen shoulder." If you ask the culture, "Where does it hurt?" one of the places the culture hurts is in areas of body shame, eating, and body size because it's a social issue: a gender issue related to sexism. Seven out of eight Americans with eating disorders are women. Ninety-seven percent of all women have hateful voices in their heads about their bodies. The diet industry banks on women feeling that they're not attractive, and then they are unsuccessful on a diet and feel even more internalized hatred and shame.

The body of our culture says, "Here are my symptoms: eating, body size, body shame, diet programs that don't work. This is what you should be paying attention to." These are symptoms, but then we must investigate the deeper illness: violence, abuse, systemic cultural sexism, and relationship problems—all are issues pointing arrows at a cultural pandemic. Sexual violence can trigger significant, swift weight fluctuations. Weight can show up as a form of protection against sexual violence. When I work with just one woman, I often see all these things—a world view —but happening on the inside.

What does it look like to talk to her and not think she's "screwed up," to respect that person and think her body is responding in intelligent ways? If a woman hasn't been educated, especially by other women, she won't be thinking about her body in terms of outer world issues, nor as part of a body of a culture that's suffering.

What people call fat-shaming is still one of the most acceptable kinds of humor, although it's becoming less so. Women are expected to laugh along with fat jokes, not say "Ouch." Many don't feel like they have permission to come out and say, "That was a rude joke." They turn it inward and ask, "What's wrong with me that I can't take a joke?" Women don't often have a boundary or a defense system around themselves in that area. This dominant paradigm is in the air we breathe.

In this book, that paradigm is not dominant. It exists and I acknowledge it, but I propose another paradigm entirely. How can you get from there to here? Paradigm shifts are both simple and difficult. If you get the shift, it's like, *Oh! The world is round!* And suddenly your belief that the world is flat is gone for good. But if everyone around you still believes the world is flat, it's easy to lose sight of your epiphany. What makes the paradigm so difficult to shift? We're working with embedded views, presumptions.

The dominant paradigm is, "I look at myself and I see so much I don't like. I'll try to change it, and look for ways to do that." People search for gurus, programs, blog posts, coaches, all coming from an allopathic place, as if size is a sickness that needs a cure. Then the program doesn't work, and people feel like failures. But if ninety-five percent of people aren't successful, something's wrong with this whole thing.

In the allopathic model, "What I don't like about myself should be removed in some way, to get rid of the problem." On a global scale, getting rid of "the Jewish Problem" led to genocide. It's the same mindset. It's deadly. It kills people. When people die of eating disorders, they have hated themselves to the point of not living.

There's another paradigm: I think all kinds of colors, shapes, and aspects have their own intelligence. Bees, bats, ice—everything has a natural intelligence that works together with everything else. A better world would be friendly, celebratory toward all of that. When I work with clients, I think, "Just like nature, your body is doing something that, like any other kind of diversity, has intelligence and beauty." But it's hard to get through to people because they're so imbued with the dominant paradigm. And they want to prove they're correct.

We need a diversity model, one that seeks to understand and celebrate the beauty and intelligence in all shapes and sizes.

I ask, "What is that person hungry for?" Are they looking for sweetness when they crave sweets? Spiciness because their life is too bland? To feel ecstatic? There's intelligence in the diversity of nature, and people seek diversity in their food. And they may have gotten bigger to protect themselves. Let's celebrate the intelligence of that protectiveness.

Acknowledging the intelligence, beauty, and moral correctness of an individual's body restores power and grace. Getting over fixing ourselves means getting over a kind of violence that's been internalized for generations.

In the following chapters, you'll witness the powerful transformations of seventeen women who collaborated with me on this work. They brought their bodies and unconscious hungers outside the shame fortress and into the light of awareness. And nothing was ever the same again.

Chapter One

Alexis: *The Joy of "No!"*

~

*"When you say no, it's about agency, independence, personhood.
You have to see me as a person. I'm me."*

ALEXIS TELLS A universal woman's story. Like almost all diet stories, it begins with her rejection of her body as it is: "too big," and an obstacle, she thinks, to finding love. It is a story of the intention to diet, followed by rejection of the plan she intended to follow—the ideals that moved her to diet and the rejection of the criticism they imply.

I begin with her story because she so clearly and unabashedly describes a fundamental underlying dilemma that most dieters face: if the diet program is not aligned with your deeper needs and nature, then you will sabotage it, derail it, resist it, and ensure that it fails. Alexis describes it this way: "Whenever I even think about starting a diet program, all of a sudden I start consuming foods that I don't consume, on a daily basis, in greater amounts. I feel like I'm starving to death. It's crazy. And this happens before I even officially go on the diet. To be fighting it when I'm not even in a program seems crazy to me, but that's what happens. I decide I'm going to have salad every day, or drink this much water, but then I start reaching for the snacks. I find myself eating chocolate—and I don't even like chocolate!"

While this pattern does not always appear in such an obvious form, it's what's behind a lot of repetitive dieting—a pattern you will see in other stories.

Alexis opened my eyes to the power of saying no to dieting, to the life force behind not following a program. Who among us has not been asked to follow a program that twisted us, contorted us, misshaped us, without sufficient regard for the truth of who we really are, our feelings or esteem? Who has not been evaluated, critically, coldly, even harshly by people with eyes blind to our deeper beauty, gifts, and intelligence? Who has not been asked to live in a smaller space than our spirits would willfully inhabit? (I recall the genie in the movie *Aladdin*, played brilliantly by Robin Williams, who emerged from his magical lantern home, reflecting what his life was like: "Phenomenal cosmic power, itty bitty living space.") When our greatness is not seen, sometimes we insist on being seen via that which is impossible to ignore: our bodies.

When weight-loss programs fail to note and address this issue, they become complicit in a culture of misogyny, aligning with the insidious viewpoint that women should be quieter, smaller—invisible.

A Brief History: There's No Diet Without Love

Alexis is thirty-two years old, a single mother of two children, an overweight woman in a family of overweight women, from her great-grandmother on down.

Alexis says her mother had always been heavy, heavier than any of her friends' moms. Her mother tried to lose weight and went on diets that worked, for a while. But then she would gain it all back again. "She was so frustrated," Alexis said. "Now my mom doesn't do anything about it. She sits around and really doesn't move any more than she has to."

When I ask her what she wants to tell her mother, Alexis says, "Get off your butt! You do these things to yourself, things that kill you, like smoking and being overweight. If I don't fix this, that's where I'll be in thirty years." Alexis sees a future she doesn't want, but doesn't see her mother, like her, up against misogynistic forces.

When Alexis was a child, her peers made fun of her. She never felt like the prettiest girl. "People didn't like me. My best friend was prettier, skinnier, taller, but maybe that was just in my head. Still, I'm thirty-two, and no one wants to date me."

Most people on a diet can easily summon painful moments: the tandem blows of insensitive and brutal comments spoken by others, and their own shame-soaked inner criticism.

Sustainable dieting often requires a more loving foundation than anyone might think. Too often, diet programs begin without sufficient heart, understanding, and compassion. The weight-loss agenda overrides the need for our pain to be noted, felt, and witnessed with a warm heart, a patient ear, and a compassionate eye.

Weight-loss agendas rarely speak of rape and the assault on women's bodies, psychology, and spirituality.

While one part of us may insist on a cut-and-dried diet plan, another part often insists on being treated with respect and love. This is the healthy part of us that wants to stick up for ourselves against external and internalized criticism, the part of us that continues to argue with someone in our heads, to make them see, to win, hours after the exchange has ended. To win—not just for the sake of winning—but to win the love we deep-down feel we deserve.

We all know the tenacity, the force of this voice, because we try to shut it off, and then there it is again, a couple of minutes later. This force alone is enough to sidetrack any diet plan. No matter how much we try to change ourselves by the numbers on the scale, most of us simply won't trade a smaller number for less love, whether we are aware of this dynamic or not. Our frustration grows with each seeming failure. It's a vicious cycle with one under-the-radar saving grace: our demand for love stands victorious.

Alexis grew up watching her mother fail at dieting, and at the same time, she endured her father's unchecked perfectionism. As an adult, she is faithful to her parents in that she has the same weight struggles as her mother, and the strict, perfectionistic outlook of her father.

"With my father, when things aren't together, you better stand clear. He doesn't even say hello—he immediately starts in." She recalls his parenting style as punishing and hurtful. She admits she sometimes parents her children the same way. "I lose control of myself, and start yelling and screaming." She says she wants her kids to be excited to see her, not to shut down in the face of her scoldings. Screaming because everything isn't perfect just fosters feelings of futility. Why bother, when it'll never be good enough? "Just because things are messy, you don't have to lose control of your head."

Harnessed fruitfully, this perfectionism could power any change Alexis put her mind to, but without tempering, it lacks compassion and love. When Alexis even thinks about beginning a diet plan, her inner father shows up to do it "perfectly," and she slips right into rebellious resistance—because she's a grownup now, and she can claim her power without being punished by him. Yet it's still problematic and self-defeating: eating in a way that goes against her goals and wishes. She feels her rebellion defeats her; she does not yet know that her rebellion is not the problem, it's the solution.

Whenever a fierce and powerful motivation to change arises in Alexis, she valiantly zeroes in on a diet program and begins to take it on with fervor and strong intention. However, because these diet plans are by the numbers, devoid of love and compassion, complicit in her oppression, they agree with the criticizers who haunt her self-esteem. And so, because she resists being hurt, refuses to shrink, she will also refuse or resist the diet program. She thinks she's eating illogically, but it makes perfect sense. She's trying to chew her way out of the trap of judgment and self-loathing.

I ask Alexis, "If you were confident, really confident about dieting, what would you do differently?"

"I would set up an exercise schedule, have people go with me, surround myself with people who are health-oriented, stick to it. But I don't know how strict I would be with the food." She laughs. "I don't like measuring food, it makes me more hungry. When I think I can only have this food or that food, I suddenly really want all the things that I shouldn't eat. 'Mmm, look at that candy bar over there.' I don't even like sweets, but all of a sudden, I am craving sweets."

"Tell me more about wanting to rebel."

"I can have a little bit of this, a little bit of that. I don't have to write that down, even if I'm keeping a food journal. I am going to show you I have power."

"What is your power like? You said you are going to show me your power, let's see it."

"I'm not going to eat all of your carrots. I'll stick to your plan most of the way, but not totally."

"You're not going to stick to my plan, exactly," I say, joining her in a role play.

"I would like to, but I can't. No matter how hard, how badly I want to stay right inside this box, I can't." Her perfectionism and self-criticism conflict with her rebellion and desire to claim her power.

"But you have to," I say, playing the role of the diet. "These are my rules and you must stick within them. I don't want you to mess around. I made plans that are good for you, I don't want you squeezing out."

"I can't, I just can't. I have to be able to—" she laughs. Alexis's smiles, giggles, and laughter betray that she takes pleasure in her rebellion.

This kind of dialogue with one's diet program, the rules and philosophy, is often essential if we are to become more aware of the yo-yo dieting dynamic: one that can almost never be overcome. Instead of chasing the rhythm of losing and gaining and losing weight, all the while feeling increasing shame and hopelessness, we can unearth and investigate this dynamic and reap the rewards of its deeper intelligence.

"I don't get to say no very often. With my kids I sometimes get to say no, and I love it."

"Teach me about the importance of saying no. You are the guru of saying no. Teach me the joy of no."

"It's getting to put your two feet on the ground and say no. It's just for you, it's only for you. It's the ability to say those words and have no repercussions. You can't do it at work, because you can't afford to lose your job. If I say no in the places where I can,

I'll be able to hold back from saying it in the places where I can't."

Of course, the one place Alexis *can* say no is to her diet plan. While her conscious goal is to diet, her unconscious goal is equal to and contrary to dieting. In a way, Alexis sets up the perfect place to practice her deeper, yet unconscious, developmental goal: learning to resist, to say no.

"Dear Ms. No, it seems there are areas in life where you would also like to say no, but the costs are too great. You're a single mom. You really need to keep your job."

"That's true."

"But you still get to exercise your no where you can."

"When I say no, it gives me the ability to recognize myself. My own wants, my own feelings, it's everything about me. Everything stops. This is about me, I'm doing this for me, I'm saying no because I can, I am saying no because I don't want to, I am saying no because of me. Everything else in life is about my family, my job, my bills, my friends who need me. It's about society, charity, everything. I have to give. Give, give, give. No one ever turns around and looks at me and asks what I need as a person."

I think, "Thank goodness she has found a place to assert herself, even though it undermines her diet plan." I find myself almost rooting for the part of her who eats when she plans to diet; I certainly root for her standing up for herself. She is singing a song for herself, just herself. Can you hear the music?

This discovery, this insight, is of profound importance to almost every one of us who seeks to change something about ourselves. While we set out upon the path to our stated goal, just under the surface there often lies a contrary desire, an oppositional dedication, and an antithetical logic!

Entering into a diet program without knowing your inner goal is a path to failure. Worse, it is often a path to further self-condemnation and shame.

"It's a very beautiful relationship you have with eating," I observe. "It's a safe place, a place to say something fundamental: 'This is me, I'm here.' It's gorgeous. Right in the middle of this place we're calling dieting, one part of you says, 'Plow right through, you have the power to do it,' but in that same dieting place, right there, someone barely speaks, saying, 'This is the place where I get to take a very basic stance, where I declare, "I'm here." It's so fundamental that I almost don't exist without it. If you don't understand that, and try to take that from me, you will be making a grave error.' I never heard anyone talk about dieting the way you are."

She beams and shines. "I never talked this way before now."

To Alexis, eating a snack is a "no" to a certain life that is not only without agency and power, but a life she feels she must live, a life with priorities and values she does not agree with.

Following No to Infinite Yes

Our dialogue now goes deeper, beyond rebellion to the core of Alexis's being. She begins talking about her children. "When they say no, it's about their agency, their independence, their very personhood. It's like, 'No, I am not a baby, you have to see me as a person. I'm me.' There has to be a safe place where they can say no. As adults too, we need a safe place."

"When you say 'me,' what are you referring to?"

"It's that comfortable part of myself. I don't need to be anything for anybody else. Everything slows down, your brain slows down, you don't have to achieve anything in that moment.

It's all about you. There is nothing to be achieved, there is no-where you have to go. It's like leaning back in your chair and taking a really deep breath and then just exhaling extremely slowly. And when you exhale, you release everything you have to do, everything everyone is expecting of you. The only thing left to get done is what you want to do, and at this moment you don't want to do anything."

"But what about all the things I have to do? There are so many things I have to get done in a day," I ask, challenging Alexis to strengthen her resolve in getting this need met.

"All of those things will just fall into place, they always do. Maybe not the way you think they should fall into place, but it will fall into place. You let go long enough to reset who you are. It's like that moment when you are just waking up. You are not thinking yet about what you have to get done."

Alexis is describing something closer to a spiritual state: a state of being where there is neither something to do nor a re-bellion. Cultivating this resting place will be key to her future efforts to diet and to feel well through life's vicissitudes.

Her insights remind me of my years of studying and prac-ticing meditation. As she shares this wisdom, it seems as if she has been studying and teaching mindfulness for years. This is the center from which one can reinvent oneself and make the deeper life changes that the body issues are just a symbol for.

"If you could go back, what kind of life would you build if you started out with this wisdom?"

"It would be a lot less structured, I would put things in a different order. Family time should be more abundant, and working shouldn't take as much time. It should be completely reversed from how the culture actually is."

First I thought Alexis's saying "no" was a kind of resistance to get over. Then I learned it was an expression of agency, of power, of selfhood. That would have been important enough. But now I am learning that saying "no" is more than that; it is a doorway into breathing, stopping the world, resetting, and a realignment of values and what is of value. It is the beginning of her turning her lived priorities on their head.

"I can give a lot, but something has to be given back to me. We can put out a lot more than what we take in. But we need to be replenished, and if there is nobody else to give it to you, then you have to give it to yourself. People place their value on their actions. There's more to you than your actions. You are always something more than what you can give to someone else."

I thanked Alexis for sharing her teaching with me.

"Thank you," she says. "It becomes real once it is said aloud."

Alexis left me with a newfound respect and awe for the human capacity for creativity. In her seemingly disturbing habit of eating more as soon as she decided to diet grew the seed of her power, deeper values, and spirit. Alexis was not only saying "no" to a diet plan that was too superficial for her to really and fully sign on to, she was also saying "no" to the world of action, to outer evaluation, and to giving herself away. She was saying yes to her own needs, her own values, her own spirit, her own self.

When I began studying mindfulness meditation, I learned that the meditations I was learning were not initially taught to lay people (referred to as "householders"), or women for that matter. It was thought that the teaching was for monks and really couldn't be integrated into the everyday life of work, family, and relationships. Only the monks could really dedicate themselves to "stopping the world." This changed when several men and women teachers in the mid-twentieth century began teaching retreats for lay folk. Now I see that whether it was taught to lay folk or not, the human spirit, in its inexorable power and capacity for creative manifestation, still finds a way to practice, even if it is in the eating of a piece of chocolate.

Or as that wonderful meditation teacher and writer Stephen Levine said, echoing the wisdom of the Japanese tea ceremony, "Taking a cup of tea, I stop the war."

Chapter Two

Anna: *Fitting In*

"I could go away and die and no one would notice.
It wouldn't even matter."

WEIGHT LOSS IS tied up with fitting into clothing, whether at home or in a dressing room—the skinny jeans, the fat pants, that dress in the window.

Is it more than a play on words that *fitting in* with other humans is also important? Anna's story is about not fitting in, as a person, as a girl, and as a woman. Her feelings of exclusion are at the root of the pain she has suffered her whole life, from her parents, to the "in" groups in school, to her adult family and work life.

"I was always trying to appease people," she says. Part of fitting in is hiding the parts of yourself that you think will prevent you from being accepted and included, and Anna, like so many of us, got used to presenting less and less of herself.

This is what Anna's story is about: the conflict between her desire to feel accepted socially, and to be her own person in a family and culture with beliefs that work against female sovereignty, power, and leadership. Carl Jung and others say that this conflict certainly shows up in dreams. Arny Mindell and others have noted that these conflicts also express themselves somatically, showing up in the body. Our bodies are intelligent, powerful, and expressive entities, formed by biochemistry, the choices we make, as well as the feelings we suppress. One of the many ways the body expresses itself is through size and weight.

Our bodies may not conform to the attitudes and standards we consciously value. They may not fit in. In that way, they may be expressing parts of ourselves that have been suppressed.

In junior high, Anna's body got bigger while her friend, who has a slighter frame, remained thin. "Why is this happening to me and not you?" she asked her friend, while her inner shame, the sense that something was wrong with her, remained unseen in the background.

Parts of Anna were not free to feel and respond because shame was suppressing them. Because going back to earlier events and recovering those feelings is a healing direction, I ask Anna to close her eyes and imagine herself in grade school. How does she feel?

"I feel fat," Anna says.

"What does that mean?" I ask, curious. "Do you feel heavy, bloated, a sense of having overeaten?"

"No, I feel badly about myself." Anna doesn't describe her body, but how she feels about it.

"What does it feel like to feel fat?" I question further.

"I don't feel accepted," she says.

Anna's sensation of feeling fat registers to her in the context of others' perspectives, attitudes, and actions. I want to focus on her feelings as something apart from the criticism she has internalized. Many people with body image issues can't differentiate between their own feelings about themselves and the attitudes and behaviors of others. Their actual feelings get lost, which takes away their ability to navigate from an authentic place.

"How did you feel when kids made hurtful comments?"

"I felt hurt and angry. I told myself, 'I don't look good.' I wanted to look like someone else. As a young girl, self-esteem is so huge. If you feel good, you have better conversations. If you don't feel good, then you act differently. I became introverted. I didn't do a lot of things because I didn't feel good. I remember thinking, 'I wish I had those clothes, I wish I could sit in that moment and have a good conversation and fit in the group.'" She quickly moves on from feeling hurt and angry to what she tells herself.

"What does 'fitting in' mean to you?"

"Having a fun personality. I envied my peers who were athletic, outgoing, and always had a group of friends who wanted to spend time with them."

"Did you try to conform in an effort to fit in?"

"I would give in to some degree. But then I would start to think, 'Why would I let these people dictate so much?' Unfortunately, social groups really affect us a lot. I really wanted to feel accepted and appreciated, to be told that I was a good friend, a good person, and that I was doing good things," she explains. "This also tied into my family dynamic. I always felt that my younger brother had those kinds of friends. When I was in about fifth grade, my father was a coach. Even though I played sports too, he mostly coached my younger brother. He put a lot of energy into my brother, not me. I don't think my father even realized how involved he was with coaching my brother. My mom was the same way."

"So your brother was in the 'in' group in your family, and you were excluded from that intimacy. This pattern re-created itself in your social life."

"Yes, it made me feel like I didn't matter." The hurt and

anger was less available to her when she was a child and simply felt badly about herself.

As an adult, Anna is also used to feeling like she doesn't matter. When someone, often her husband, puts her down, she's so used to it that she has become blind to it. We become inured to inner and outer criticism when we are shamed for our feelings and reactions to it when we are young. Instead, we take up the mission of trying to change ourselves, to fit in more.

"My husband will say, 'Are you going to wear those shorts? They don't look good on you.'" As Anna tells me about her husband's comments, again she doesn't seem to notice how hurtful they are. I ask her how her husband's comment makes her feel.

"Well, it makes me distant."

"What do you want to say to him?"

"I know I need to do some things to change, but your comment about my shorts doesn't support positive change." She's getting closer to her authentic reaction.

However, as we talk more about it, she shares that she is trying to develop a thicker skin, still thinking it is she that should change, alter herself, fit in with her husband's attitudes. Because she is willing to put up with a kind of abuse, not free to assert herself, she thinks she should get tougher.

"What happens when your husband says, 'You don't really look good in those shorts'?"

"My feelings get hurt. How dare you say I look bad? It cuts me down. It makes me feel little. I feel little, less of a person." Yet her reply is matter-of-fact, without feeling.

"That's a big hurt," I point out. "Help me connect with that experience, to feel 'less of a person.'"

"Like I don't fit in. I'm not accepted for who I am. I don't meet the mark. I'm not valued."

Anna's response goes back to her core wound of not fitting in. Her voice lowers. Her statements are just that; they carry little feeling. Anna needs more contact with these feelings.

"'I don't matter,'" I say. "Is that it?"

She nods. "I could go away and die and no one would notice. It wouldn't even matter. Why should I do anything? I'm not part of anything, part of the group. I don't really matter. This is big. I never really thought about it."

For Anna, not fitting in is connected to feeling isolated and shunned, as in childhood. Far from a feeling that she can dismiss or bypass by wanting to get tougher, these experiences make her imagine dying. While I wasn't worried about literal suicidality, this kind of statement needs to be taken deadly seriously. It indicates that she can disappear in relationship, not speak the words in her heart, and suffer from a lack of connection with her very life force—a kind of background depression. But now she's an adult and can reengage with the world around her more powerfully. She just needs to experience a paradigm shift from the shame of thinking she needs to fit in or get tougher, to being in touch with and valuing her feelings and reactions.

In an effort to help Anna further make this shift, I engage in a role play.

"If you were this 'in crowd' person criticizing yourself, what would you say?"

"I'd say, 'You are not good enough. You can go ahead and eat because you are not going to stick with dieting—or anything else you try. So why bother?'"

I notice the connection between her inner critic and her eating decisions. She gives herself the message that it's okay to take pleasure from food, but only because nothing she does actually matters.

Often, when a person gets more in touch with early stories, other stories with similar dynamics from the past and present arise. She recounts what happened when she was assaulted at work.

"I worked in a youth correctional facility. I was hit in the face and the head. I was transported in an ambulance to the hospital." She gives her report in a singsong voice, like the incident was nothing. She uses the passive voice. She doesn't refer to the attacker directly. She's not yet in touch with her feelings and reactions.

"What did you get hit with?"

"A fist, a two-by-four of some kind. Yeah, I needed some oral surgery." She delivers the information with an air of nonchalance. "It was pretty traumatic, but I felt like I didn't matter." Again, the sense of "not mattering" surfaces, erasing her experience, and erasing her.

"The one person I wanted to be there wasn't there," she says, her disconnection showing up in the way she doesn't name her husband.

It is clear that she is being assaulted, internally and externally. Someone might have seen the assault at her job. But when she beats herself up, there are no witnesses. No one is there to say, "You matter," or even "You exist," which would counteract the deadliness of this dynamic.

Stepping Out

I am wanting to see if Anna has a life force in her that can counter the annihilating force of inner and outer critics. This is the medicine she needs.

"What is the opposite of not mattering?" I ask.

"Being selfish and arrogant," she says.

These qualities are part of Anna's shadow; they are split off and marginalized by her usual personality. Yet she needs the essence of these qualities to combat the shame and recover her deeper self.

"Show me that experience," I tell her. "Let's feel what it would be like to be selfish and arrogant."

"It's all about me. I am the priority. You figure out your stuff because I have my agenda. Everything is about me, you people are not that important to me." It's a great sign that she can generate this so readily. Many people will simply become silent or insist that being selfish and arrogant is not a good thing, thus suppressing their life force.

"Yes," I say, reflecting back her thoughts. "I don't think about others so much. They are not important to me." This is what she needs to integrate.

"And I don't really care about what others have to say, because I am going to do what I am going to do anyway," she continues.

"Keep telling me about this kind of person," I say in order to help her stay in touch with the medicine she needs to heal her shame.

"It's all about me. I have things I want to do, and I am cut-throat. No one will get in my way."

"Yes, you are on a mission," I say, affirming her words. "If people get in your way, you take them down. You don't hate them, they are just in your way."

"Right, I don't have to consider others."

Some people should never be told, "Stop caring about what others think, feel, or need," but when a person follows the dictate to fit in and accommodate, then "not caring" about others is just the right medicine—a form of stepping out.

"What would you do if you could be that person?"

"I would be career-driven. I would go places where things are worthy of me."

"You think you belong there, don't you? What's so great about you?" I ask, playing devil's advocate.

"I am a competent person, I have integrity and respect. I can do anything I need to, to get things done. I am very truthful and committed. I generally want to see good things happen. I can also say the hard things."

Anna truly fits in somewhere: a place where her career and the people around her are worthy of the caliber of person she actually is! Anna also shows leadership qualities. I further the dialogue to see if she can also claim this part of herself, to support her in finding a fit being more of a leader than a follower.

"You're a leader."

"I want to be one. I don't see myself as that," she says with a smile.

"Why do you smile?"

"Because I don't have the confidence to be a leader."

"Let's forget the confidence," I suggest. "Let's go back to your selfishness." The sense of selfishness is where Anna contacts her shadow-self, which is where her confidence lies.

"I have a bigger picture of how things should be. The challenge is that I get frustrated. I often have to dumb things down so that my coworkers understand me. I don't want to have to do that."

"Tell me about being so far ahead."

"It's frustrating, I don't have the patience."

"What are you thinking about those people?"

"I think they are incompetent." *There it is.* "I am not putting them down, they are just not competent."

One part of Anna is still hung up on fitting in. She doesn't want to confront people or put them down; she'd rather follow others, fit in, and get along with them. Another part has no impulse to fit in; she's a leader, ahead of others.

"But doesn't a little part of you want to say, 'I want to challenge these people'?" That's what a leader does when they feel ahead of others.

"Yeah, about fifty percent of me."

That's half of her—more than the little part she spoke of earlier.

"What would it say?"

"You need to move forward. Challenge yourself."

This part of Anna doesn't care about following and fitting in. She matters to herself. She trusts her own opinions enough to see her own worth without waiting for people to tell her she's good enough to fit in. Her own deeper feelings and reactions, previously suppressed, bring her home to herself. It is quite the opposite of how she is used to experiencing herself.

She smiles and feels an unfamiliar joy—being in her internal "in crowd." She is a leader, not a follower. She won't try to fit in just as her body won't fit in—amen. She has integrated some of her body intelligence. I sit with Anna and feel in her a new sense of ease.

Chapter Three

Vanessa: *Loving the Bear*

~~~

"In the army, I used to rub a mad amount of hemorrhoid cream
around my ass and thighs and wrap myself in Saran Wrap,
because it shrinks tissues. I could hang with the guys,
I could do what I was supposed to do, but my ass was too big."

VANESSA GAVE ME a deep understanding of what it's like when arbitrary measurements are applied to a person without their consent. You may be in excellent health, you may be able to pass every fitness test, but all that is nullified if your hip measurements exceed a random number.

In Vanessa's case, she bumped up against the U.S. military's body measurement rules, but these rules are an extreme example of the way women in our culture who don't fit into the petite female aesthetic are abused by institutions and norms.

Patriarchal dogma decrees that men are big and strong, and women are delicate and fine-boned. Women are even allowed to be strong, as long as they aren't too big. Regardless of this outdated belief, strong women come in all shapes and sizes.

Many women who judge themselves as bigger than a fictional norm spend significant time and energy trying to make themselves small, without taking the time to question whether what is driving them is valid.

Over the course of her life, Vanessa encountered "little things": put-downs and statements about how she *should* be—

smaller, more petite. This conflicted with her inner truth: she liked her size, enjoyed her strength. Vanessa was told by everyone, from her father to the U.S. military, that she wasn't acceptable because she didn't fit into a belief based on sexist wishful thinking. When everyone around you is telling you something untrue, it can cause you to question and distrust yourself, which introduces shame. It can also siphon off valuable energy to argue back, either verbally or in your own head. (Think of all of the better uses for that energy!)

Vanessa was not only physically a big woman, she also had a big spirit. Once I understood this, my goal was to reunite Vanessa with her bigness in a way that would allow her to embrace and celebrate herself the way she was, without shame and internalized disapproval.

When I met Vanessa, she was struggling with whether to take the firefighter test. She was also studying to be a paramedic and was worried about whether she should continue. She worried that maybe it was the wrong path, that it was just too much.

When we begin talking about her weight, she admits, "This is not something I have ever talked about." As she tells me more about her life story, it seems more and more poignant that she had absorbed so many negative messages about her body without ever allowing herself to ask others for a reality check, most likely because her feelings of shame questioned her experience, leaving her doubting her truth.

Vanessa first became aware of body image and body weight when she was in elementary school, around age seven or eight. These early moments of coming to consciousness around one's body can lock in beliefs, internalized criticism, and shame for years to come.

"My father was talking to his friends in the yard, and I

heard him say, 'Yep, she is a husky girl.' That really stood out to me. I felt more defensive than anything. I know I'm not a petite girl, but what's wrong with that?" she asks. "It was a funny description. I didn't identify with it. And luckily, it took me a long time to realize that it's 'not okay' to be a big girl, full-framed, full-figured, big-boned, whatever you want to call it. There was a time when that wasn't part of my awareness, and then it was."

Even though it was not part of Vanessa's awareness, the message entered her psyche, creating a conflict between her true self, who was big in spirit, and a viewpoint that was critical, urging her to be smaller. It's like waking up in a house that isn't yours and being accused of trespassing. You find yourself in the wrong without having done anything wrong. And then shame's repetitive self-talk takes it one deadly step further, from "You are in the wrong" to "You are wrong; wrong is what you are."

"When I was thirteen, I was the tallest in my class, and I thought that was cool. I'm five-foot-nine, but when I put some boots on—" She strikes a proud pose. I can see and feel, viscerally, the innate truth express itself in her body's movements, the strength of her desire to feel good in her skin.

"When I was that age, there was some joke about my weight, and I said, 'I am the same weight as Cindy Crawford.' And my friend's mother said, 'Yeah, but how tall is she?' I felt good enough about myself to say, 'There's nothing wrong with me.'"

"But indirect comments like that are insidious," I say.

"It's the little stuff that adds up," she says. "Maybe eventually you give in to it. I have only been overweight, officially, for about four years. Now I feel fat, I wasn't fat before. I was big, but not fat. I was like, 'This is okay, this is the way I am,' and that was the attitude I was pushing out there."

She needed to "push it out there," to devote force to a

protective, defensive energy, just to stand her ground, to stay still. She wants to inhabit her big and tall self, but there are forces against her that prevent her from resting in that acceptance and celebration.

"I can now look back at pictures and think, 'Man, did I look great.'" She says this with pride, passion, and verve, pushing the statement out there. "But that's not what I felt like then. I felt big, like I do now. And not in a good way."

Vanessa's experience is consistent with many women I have worked with who always felt too big, but when they look at earlier photos, they see it wasn't true. Their experience of being "too big" resulted from internalized views of those around them. Their eyes were not their own; instead, they wore the culture's glasses, along with the attitudes, preferences, even the disgust and contempt that went along with them.

"I have broad shoulders, a big ribcage, big legs. I never felt like I was where I was supposed to be. I was always too big, always ten pounds too heavy. It is just out of reach, never quite there. It's like tying your shoe when the gun goes off," she laughs. As Vanessa talks in the presence of a witness, she makes more contact with how ever present the assault on her body and psyche were. Some part of her "always" felt too big.

Vanessa is telling me, through her analogy, that she is ready and able to run a race, to take on something big, but this truth is undermined by the belief that she needs to be smaller. That belief doesn't see her readiness, her power, her capacity. In fact, it denigrates these qualities as less feminine, something to shed. That is what ties her up. In a way, it's true; she's not ready when the gun goes off, but it's not because she is too heavy, it's because she is carrying around the weight of a belief that doesn't belong to her. It's that belief, not her weight, that she needs to shed.

"It's that I'll never be exactly who I am supposed to be, part of the group. When I think back on all my friends in high school, or in the Army, I wanted to be a part of those groups, but they always saw me as not quite there. But I am there, dammit," she pushes out. "I don't see the boundary."

I bring her back to that early story—her first memory of that belief entering her psyche. "I am thinking of your dad and his friend, 'She's a husky girl.'"

"There are a million things he could have said about me. It's a put-down, it was underhanded. He could have said, 'She's powerful, there's something amazing about her, she's unstoppable.' And a guy can be husky, but a girl... it took away my femininity or something. I don't know."

"If you were a guy, he would have called you *strong*. You're just like one of the guys, but not."

She is quiet, then shares, "In the military, you have to be tape-tested. You have to fit into their little body mass index chart. Well, as a woman," she laughs, "as a *curvy* woman, you're screwed. I was supposed to be 156 pounds or something ridiculous, at five-foot-nine. If you are not under that weight, they have to tape you and measure you. They do all these measurements around your wrist, around your forearm, around your neck and your *ass*," she says with a special sarcasm. "And they enter the measurements into an equation and they say, 'You're too fat.' They would say this, independent of whether I passed all of the physical tests."

"Like, 'Well, you're strong enough, you can do all the tests, but your ass is too big.'"

"Exactly, it's infuriating, it's ridiculous. And then you get put on remedial physical training. During my whole four years in the Army, I went back and forth between being too fat and just barely squeaking by. I used to rub a mad amount of hemorrhoid cream around my ass and thighs and wrap myself in Saran Wrap, because it shrinks tissues. And I am not the only one who did that. Seriously," she sighs, totally exasperated. "It's ridiculous. I could put on a 5-10 tire by myself. I could hang with the guys, I could do what I was supposed to do, but my ass was too big. It's so embarrassing to have to go to remedial PT. It's humiliating, they call it 'fat camp.' My sergeants would say, 'Why are *you* here?' because I could clearly do everything I was supposed to be able to do. On top of that, it's constantly held over your head when it comes to rank and promotion. I did horrible things to my body. I took pills, like ephedrine, that sped up my heart rate. I would have asthma attacks, but I am not asthmatic."

"Just to get your weight down," I say.

Even with regard to losing weight, she is fierce, unstoppable. Even in her diet approach, she manifested her power. But instead of this power showing up in the outer world and being appreciated, it showed up in her discipline to lose weight. So many women use great inner resources trying to lose weight and then resist losing weight. Can you imagine if those resources were unleashed on their relationships and the world around them?

An Abuse of Power

An additional cost of women's power being applied to diet efforts is the impact of enduring the shame and self-hatred that impels women to try to make themselves smaller. But they usually can't. Their size manifests anyway, despite their efforts and intentions. It's this conflict that we now turn to.

"Tell me about how it feels to be subject to these ideas about your size."

"My weight has been an underlying current my whole life. It's a pull, a drag."

As you saw earlier, the weight Vanessa is talking about is the weight of the struggle, not the actual physical weight.

"OK, give me a physical experience of the drag," I say. "Pull me down, drag me. Grab my hands." I'm wanting Vanessa to make a tangible physical experience of the 'drag' she is speaking about, allowing me to engage directly with her inner conflict.

She laughs. "Well, I would probably pull you to the ground."

"OK, do it slowly, so I can feel the drag." She laughs the laugh of someone who not only *knows* she could overpower me but the laugh of someone who is expressing herself outside of her comfort zone by showing me that she can overpower me. She starts to pull me. "I get it," I say. She laughs.

Not wanting her concern for me to stop her from going even further with her self-expression, I say, "Keep doing that, forget about who you are, forget about Vanessa. Your life intention is to do this, that's it."

"It's like a bear or a lion, something completely overpowering. There's so much depth, so much weight, there's so much... I'm not awake to it entirely, does that make sense?"

This is a gorgeous moment. Vanessa is not only inhabiting her full self, but relishing it, enjoying it. This kind of experience, when witnessed without shame, can change the course of a person's relationship with themselves, as well as the course of their life.

"It makes so much sense. Let's play more. Imagine being that bear, feel the strength of that, the depth, the weight."

"They are so heavy, so massive, so strong."

She bends down, and her leg muscles visibly engage.

"I like what you did with your body, bending down. Feel that massive power in you, in your legs."

"I'm not afraid of anything," she says. "It's aggressive and destructive."

"But blocking the bear's path is an attitude that says, 'She should be shrink-wrapped.' That bear should take ephedrine and use hemorrhoid cream," I say.

"It's a dragging weight," she says, exasperated. "If I were to have that strength, and use that strength to move forward—"

She laughs and stands with a great power, hands on her hips.

"Feel the bear in you again," I say. "If I were you, and you were this bear, what advice would you give me?" I address the bear: "Dear Vanessa Bear, why are you here? I keep wishing to get rid of you, to be less like you. Sometimes I am not sure of myself. I am not sure if I should go take the firefighter test. I am always not quite there, ten pounds away."

Vanessa takes deep breaths as tears flow down her face.

"I have no words," she says. "I feel something."

"Don't try to shrink me down to something smaller. I won't fit," I say, trying to help her feel into it. "I need you. You don't tell a bear that its ass is too big."

"Wow, my son's name is Bjorn, which means 'brave as a bear,'" she laughs. "You mean I just have to love it. Love the bear."

"Yes, then you can stop dragging it around."

Vanessa sits with tears pouring down her face as I speak. She's been so concerned about whether to be a firefighter, a paramedic—roles that would demand all her strength. This questioning process has led her to encounter her bear nature.

Naming the Craving

As I mentioned earlier, in the background of the hunger for certain foods is a deeper hunger, a psychological or spiritual hunger. Vanessa and I begin to explore that hunger in hopes that she can get clearer about what she wants to most essentially use her power for. This is often much greater than a specific task. It's a deeper experience of a state the person is searching for, something that makes life worthwhile.

"What food do you most crave?"

"Brownies."

"What are your favorite brownies like? Do they have icing, chips in them, nuts?" The specifics are important because it helps the person make closer somatic contact with the hunger they are satisfying (in this case, the literal taste and pleasure).

"Just the chocolate. They are gooey. They can have a little crusty edge, but generally moist. Not cakey. They gotta be thick. An inch, standard brownie thick."

I can tell from the details she is sensing the hunger.

"But it's not fudge."

"No. I'm not a fudge person, that's just straight-out goo."

"What does it taste like? Let's say I don't know what a brownie is like."

"It's encompassing." She makes a motion that is big. I'm already sensing the bigness of the bear.

"If you were to make a sound, is it like *mmm*, or *MMMM*, or deeper?"

"It's like a deep grumbly giant, *fee fie foe fum*. Substantial," she says.

"What kind of person makes that noise?"

"A big person, maybe seven-foot-nine."

"That's big."

"Maybe it's a king with a drumstick. It's good to be king. You have your huge banquet table, you're dressed in velvet, you have your drumstick and brownie and it's all good."

"What is good?"

"Everything is good, everything's peaceful. Everything is taken care of."

"Yes, but it's not a margarita on the beach. It's not a light satisfaction. This is more substantial, a buffet of brownies and drumsticks. Dear king, what is the meaning of life?"

"Just to sit and be. For everything to be how it should be. To walk about your day and just feel that powerful peace. Everything is still," she says. "It's between the parentheses."

"That pause is really delicious, really substantial and satisfying," I say. "That's what that bear is going for, even in the middle of all the crazy stuff—that pause, that great satisfaction. The substantialness, the gooey, earthy, substantialness. It takes the bear to get there. This is not a 'Let's have a vacation' peace."

"I just want to cry," Vanessa says.

"Life is a substantial banquet," I say.

Vanessa's Update

When I checked in with Vanessa years later, she told me, "You were the one who kept my hope going for EMS, as I came to you at a point of almost walking away. What a mistake that would have been! I am still a volunteer medic. It is ultimately satisfying, and also a pain in the ass, but I *love it*. I also found enough bear courage inside of me to go through with my fire training, so I am a firefighter as well. Can you believe it? And I work at a water-birth clinic with midwives as advanced life-support neonatal care. I love that as well. I got a baby breathing again the other night—whew!

"I think of the things you told me often. Instead of dragging that bear around behind me, to embody that spirit, and hold that strength instead. To bear the bear, and not let the bear 'bear' down on me. It's not an easy job, but I don't want an easy job. It's the blessing and curse—they come together. I love it. I have to."

Chapter Four

Heather: *From "Okay"-ing to Healing*

~

*"I thought I was fat, but when I look back at pictures from
that time, I see a thin girl. It was an imaginary thing.
But I felt like I had to fix something."*

WHEN HEATHER SPOKE of her four family members who
died in the last year, I heard her say under her breath, "It's
going to be OK." When she described difficulties in her relationship, she insisted, "But it was really good, it was really okay."
Even when I asked her about how she felt about being forty
pounds heavier than she wanted to be, she said, "Everything is
going to be okay—my weight, and everything."

Like many of us, Heather was dealing with trauma that was
once too big to face and grapple with. Her attempt to make
things okay acted as a double-edged sword. On the one hand,
she needed to make things 'okay' in order to cope and survive.
On the other hand, one cannot truly make things okay by pushing them out of awareness or marginalizing distress. One way
this might manifest is in the form of her persistent headaches.

"Someone taught me those words, 'It'll be okay,'" she admits, "and I hung onto them and couldn't let them go."

Heather's impulse to make things okay was powerful and
persistent. It was a force that couldn't simply be quelled by telling
her, "Stop trying to fix things. Stop trying to make everything

okay." In fact, doing that would minimize the trauma she was trying to deal with, and could turn her away from her natural impulse to soothe and heal.

This reminded me of Stephen Levine, author of *Who Dies?* who said that he had a new response to that 1960s best seller, *I'm OK—You're OK*. His proposed new title: *I'm Not OK, You're Not OK, But That's OK*. Levine found a way of facing what was really not okay and still bring some okayness to the moment. Heather would also have to find her magic formula for turning her impulse to make things okay into healing medicine.

Jungian psychologist James Hillman asserted that when it comes to psychological dilemmas, the person and the problem are not so separate—or separable. Psychological dilemmas are not problems to remove like a tumor or infection, they *are* us, and we cannot get rid of *them* without getting rid of *us*. Our problems don't change, transform, gestate, or wither away and die— *we* change, or don't. The healing is not the amputation of our problem, the healing is becoming a healer. Applying Hillman's logic to Heather would mean that I would not try to get rid of her reflexive habit of fixing, but rather help her become a truer and finer fixer—a healer.

Heather's developmental question is this: How could she deepen and mature her natural impulse to bring healing so that it would not be in service of denial, but in service of making a better life and world—one that is more truly 'okay'?

The Seed of the Quest for Okayness

Is this need to make things okay a form of denial? Certainly. But at the same time, there is an inherent, great power in the *insistence* that things be okay, along with its impulse to soothe and heal. Before we can transform this reflexive response into healing power, we must first identify what inside her profoundly needs to be made okay. Has Heather sustained a primal harm that she needs to acknowledge?

"My mother was always freaking out," Heather recalls. "She was psychotic. But I don't want to say anything bad about her." I can imagine a very young Heather first employing the self-soothing chant, "It'll be okay," while her mother yelled and screamed.

"When I freak out, I bet I'm hurting my kids the same way. I can't stand it. But I can't be mad at my mom, because I'm the same way. Who's to blame, where did it start?" Again, we see the double-edged sword of Heather's "okaying"—helping her cope, but keeping her out of touch with her suffering at her mother's hands and the anger she felt deep down.

Heather tells a story, one that has stayed with her since childhood, about a dog who was about to give birth to puppies. This dog had a bad leg and would not live unless the leg was amputated, so they amputated the leg to save her and her litter. The dog survived and gave birth to her puppies, and relearned to walk by dragging one leg. The puppies, as they learned to walk, also dragged their back legs. The puppies learned by example, assuming that their mother's limitation was theirs as well, even though they had four working legs.

People remember stories like this because they resonate with their own story. We also now know about epigenetic trauma, trauma that gets carried across generations, with children and grandchildren exhibiting strategies to cope with abuse and violence that occurred before they were born. I thought of my own Jewish background and the research on how the children of Holocaust survivors carry trauma. Telling these folks to stop 'fixing' things would be insufficient and dismissive of the trauma they were born into.

Heather's healing impulse twisted and turned as it coursed through her life. At first, she turned it on herself as she tried to make her body "perfect" in order to make herself happy. Later, her healing impulse led her to the road to her religious life. And later still, this impulse fueled the maturation of her religious life, as her passion to heal became more consciously directed and loving. I had already thought of Heather as being on the healer's path. And while it was true that Heather was a wounded person looking for healing, I also came to think of her as a healer in search of a wound.

"I can see it's something inside, but I deal with it on the outside. I organize things at work, I try to be professional, I clean the house, I try to lose weight. Even my coworkers say, 'Stop, stop —it's okay, stop organizing things and worrying about things.'" She rubs her temples. "I'm worried that talking about this is going to give me a headache."

Misguided attempts at healing and expressing power can manifest in stereotypically gendered forms. Given societal pressures, women like Heather can easily sublimate their desire for deeper healing just by doing what's expected of them, from emotional labor, to housework, to dieting.

Body-Focused Fix

Heather's urge to fix herself began at the age of twelve. Not surprisingly, she focused it on her body. Her mother's perfectionist remarks contributed to this, but Heather also grew up in a culture that idealizes and privileges thin women. In a way, the pain and torment that many adolescent girls experience relative to their body image was the perfect place to now apply her undeveloped healing art. Acknowledgment of this sexist, culturally imposed standard would have to be part of any diet program that would successfully address her concerns about being overweight.

"I thought I was fat, even though I wasn't," Heather says. "When I look back at pictures from that time, I see a thin girl. It was an imaginary thing. But I felt like I had to fix *something*." Heather's experience is not uncommon. Many girls and women, especially those suffering eating disorders, see their body shape differently than any objective view.

To understand Heather better, I decide to role-play and take on the perspective of that twelve-year-old girl at the beach.

"Okay," I say, "here I am putting on a bathing suit."

"That's ugly," she says. "You look fat and ugly."

"How? My thighs, belly, the way I walk? How am I fat, how am I ugly?"

"I always see my stomach."

"Is it too big, not flat enough? Is it just that I have one?"

"Yes, and my friends used to say, 'Why are your arms so big and so strong? They are bigger than your boyfriend's!' I used to hate that part of me, I wanted to make it go away." I see how, for Heather, making things "okay" meant trying to make parts of herself go away.

Heather continued, "I was just trying to fix myself to look like those happy model girls. You can't fix the inside stuff, but you can make the outside look acceptable."

Heather fixated on trying to be a "happy model girl" before she was conscious enough to understand that she was looking at an artificial construction. Those models were being paid to act happy, and had a team of professionals at the shoot to style their clothes, hair, and makeup—and that's before the photos were Photoshopped or airbrushed of any imperfections.

As we continue to talk about it, Heather comes to understand how a sexist culture taught her to hate her body and co-opted her impulse to care for herself.

Religion as Fix

Heather was raised in a Christian household. At one point, the path of her healing and her desire to fix intersected with the road of her religious conviction.

"Once I went to this church meeting, and while I was there, every sadness, every memory in my brain was gone, and I felt so free and so happy. It was a wonderful thing. After that, everything was Jesus—left, right, front, back, everywhere—and everything *really was* okay for about ten years. It was so beautiful to share that the sadness *can* go away. God's word can make it go *whoosh*."

This ten-year period literally was a godsend. The intensity and power of her religious faith and conviction captured the force behind her desperation to fix as well as her genuine impulse to find healing. As I listen to Heather, it reminds me of those moments of grace, like when we first fall in love, that show us what is possible, give us a glimpse of what our destination might look like, and give us a reprieve from the battle—a time to rest and heal.

But this was not the final stage of Heather's path to healing or her spiritual path, because Heather had a breakdown.

"I would cry and cry. I kept asking myself, 'Did I not pray enough? What didn't I do?' Everything I thought had been washed away came back up, and it was ugly. It included all the painful things that happened during those ten years that I refused to acknowledge. I let people treat me terribly, and I said Bible verses to deal with the pain. I got really angry."

Like an oyster produces a pearl, Heather's spirituality was provoked, and created, by an irritant: trauma and the powerful urge to fix and heal. The pearl of her spiritual path was beautiful, true, and worthy, but the irritant still needed to be addressed, otherwise her desire to fix would taint the purity of her practice, mixing denial with her pure spiritual impulse. She broke down under the strain of confusing her deep love for Jesus with the powerful habit of blindly dismissing the way some people treated her, a habit she formed as a child to survive her mother. Today we see the way a turn to religion and spiritual notions can be readily accompanied by a form of spiritual bypass: claiming a temporary form of relief, via a spiritual principle, without facing and dealing with deep pain and trauma.

"The stuff that got washed away during your ten-year Jesus honeymoon, and came back up—what was that?"

"What happened between my mom and me when I was young."

Although Heather had this breakdown, she'd still come a long way. Grounded and anchored in a deepened religious faith, Heather's healing moved forward. It provided the strength, support, and love required for her to look more deeply at her pain and her anger, instead of turning away. Heather was on a healing path—one that would not only lead her up the mountain of religion, but through the land of her body.

It's What's Inside That Counts

I remember Heather's statement, "You can't fix the inside stuff, but you can make the outside look acceptable." What is this "inside stuff"? If she doesn't learn more about it, any effort to help her diet is likely to repeat the same mistake of fixing the wrong thing.

I ask her, "Do you know what it is inside that you want to address?"

"A pain and sadness that says, 'I want to be okay.'"

"Where is it inside of you? In your eyes, in your belly?"

I thought about how much I needed to facilitate Heather's own awareness as a way of training the physician inside of her. She needed to no longer rely on received biases, understandings, bypasses, and fixes. A skilled healer needs to make a more acute and informed diagnosis. Too often our pains are spoken of in such generalities; too often we simply assume we know what people are referring to. But in the interest of true healing and in the interest of true empathy, we need to be more rigorous.

"My heart is okay, my belly is okay, my spirit is okay. That's weird. It's in my brain."

Now I know where it is, but what is it? Is it a tension, a way of thinking, an exhaustion, an intensity? I remembered that earlier in our conversation, when I was asking her about her inclination to "fix," she said she was worried that she would get a headache. We must be on the right track.

"Everything is going to be okay, my weight and everything."

"What do you mean, 'It's okay'?" I echo what she spoke of earlier, "I used to think that I wasn't practicing my religion right, and that I was fat and ugly?" Although I don't want to reinforce her hurtful words, I'm repeating what she said during the role play to try to cut through her litany of "okay."

"That's exactly the way it is. I am learning to not believe those things."

"Can you believe it all the way, completely, that you aren't fat, that you aren't ugly, that you are not practicing your religion incorrectly?"

"No, there is a fear that won't let me believe that all the way. I can't let it go."

Now we are in the struggle itself as it is manifested in the moment: the sense of being okay and the belief that something is wrong with her—a battle taking place inside her head, that gives her headaches.

"Let's get to know the fear."

"I don't know how to get to know it. If I did, I would choke it by the neck and get rid of it. I would trample it under my feet in an instant. I would destroy it."

I hear the same fervor she had for her religion, for fixing herself, for hating herself, for controlling her diet. I offer her my hand, suggesting that my wrist was like a neck. She wraps her hands around it.

"I am fear," I say. "You cannot replace me, your mom had me, you have me, and you cannot get rid of me. You got rid of me for a while, but you can't get rid of me forever."

"Can't I just let it go?" Her words say one thing, but her fierce grip says something entirely different. It is as fierce as her determination to fix herself and to pray. That fierce determination belongs to her, belongs to her story, and belongs to her healing. I decide to support the firmness of her grasp rather than her seeming interest in letting go. I assert my strength and intention by moving my whole body backwards, heightening the tension of her grip.

"What are you doing?" she asks.

"I want you to move toward me, toward fear."

She instantly pulls back and away.

"I am fear pulling you toward me," I say.

"That's not happening. I've got something, I can't figure out what it is." She began twisting, making almost a growling sound. A fierceness appears in her eyes. The fear brought this out in her —this ferocity and determination.

She lets go of my wrist. Her hands drop to her sides and form two tight fists. Her hands were still expressing the essence of the grasp she previously had on my wrist, but she contained it within herself.

"I wanted to let go, but even though I did," she says, "the fear keeps coming."

Her fear is as relentless as her fight against it. They are matched.

I copy her, making fists, fierce eyes, and I growl. "What do you see?"

"You are ugly and ferocious. It's ugly, but... *totally me!*"

"Yes, it's 'totally me.' What do I need this ugly ferociousness for? Why is it here?"

"I need it to fight the fear and overtake it. It's always there, it drives everything I do."

"You are a fighter," I say.

"But I want to be a kind of princess girl," she says. It reminds me of her fixation on being "a happy model girl."

Heather is afraid that if she becomes a fighter, she will be ugly and alone. She doesn't think she can be a fighter and be attractive too. She is beginning to free herself from these cultural messages.

Heather needed to fight her fear, including the fear about how she looked. Any program chosen by that fear, designed to make her look skinnier and weaker, would be self-injurious and at odds with her ferociousness, strength, and power. It would disempower her true calling: becoming a healer. Such programs would be destined to fail.

Any diet program intelligently and lovingly designed to enrich and enhance Heather's life must align with her strength and calling, and support her fight against her fears. She grew up seeing her anger and power as ugly, and she tried to get rid of those qualities—by saying, "It's okay, it's okay"—just as she tried to diet away whatever she thought she needed to fix.

With her newfound clarity and power, I turn back to Heather's shame about her body. I ask about the forty extra pounds, and she says, unexpectedly, that she gained it because she feels better about herself, that she is more at ease with herself. She is less directed by and possessed by her fear. For Heather at this point in her development, being heavier is healthier. Gaining weight has been a path toward, not away from, her healing. Gaining weight is a cure, not a disease.

To support Heather's new perceptions and her connection with her power, I suggested that she begin lifting some weights. I picked up two barbells in my office and began to do arm curls.

"God gave me a certain strength and wants me to feel this," I say, surprised at how the words come out of my mouth unpremeditated. Heather smiles and nods. Her power is not ugly, it is not ungodly, it's *her*!

Thinking of her power as ugly has made her want to fix

what's ugly, but thinking of her power as divine will align her as a healer.

Years after we worked together, Heather sent me an email, spurred on to reconnect after taking a Systems Thinking class and being reminded of our work together.

When I met Heather, she was an adult college student pursuing a degree in human services, working her way through school as a housekeeper for Kaiser Permanente. She still works at Kaiser Permanente—as a manager in the Patient Access Department, where fifty-two people report to her. As a team, they handle the registration of over 650 patients a day, point-of-service patient payments, and reporting of all revenue. As a healer, Heather has grown to the point where she applies her fixing instincts to the smooth running of an institution focused on healing thousands of people every week. Her drive to fix supports the constituents of a healing organization with an epic scope.

Heather's titanic desire to make things okay was in fact trapped in the bubble of herself and her personal relationships, where, thus confined, it went a bit haywire. Nobody had given her a big enough problem to fix. Here we see how much a sexism that undercuts women's career ambitions can be detrimental to both individuals and to society. And its flip side—how much good is unleashed when women like Heather are able to step into their giftedness.

"All these years I have been calling it a love for resourcing. I really like seeing people come together to unravel a need, and then meet that need with things that are already available.

How big is the potential impact of her drive to heal and fix? Her closing comment gives a strong indication: "I want to map the entire world now."

Heather's Update

Just prior to this book going to press, Heather got in touch with me. She wrote, "At fifty, I have a healthy body image. I maintain an enjoyable healthy exercise routine, and continue to explore recipes and fun ways to implement vegan, vegetarian, and whole foods into my diet. My relationship with my weight and body size has transitioned to more of a focus on the overall health of my mind, body, and spirit as one, rather than a narrow view of the reflection I see in the mirror.

"Although a forever journey, learning to appreciate where worth truly comes from rather than what I must be or produce to *be* worthy has shifted a lifetime of destructive thought and behavior patterns. Thanks be to God, I have pushed passed racist assumptions of what I am or what I am not, what has been done to me or where I did not measure up. I have learned to live freely, honestly taking inventory of the masks I live behind, masks of pain, masks of abuse and protection, masks of trying to be righteous when my heart, mind, and spirit are a destructive mess. Honesty brought the next teacher as I began to realize that there was no person, formula, or substance I could cling to that would ever heal the beliefs or wrath I felt toward myself at all times. The freedom I now enjoy makes me want to dance and enjoy each moment for what it is, not what I demand it to be. It fills me with hope and expectation to see the precious promises God has prepared for us when we stop running after our own understanding, religion, opinions, and cultural checklists."

Chapter Five

Erica: *Starbucks Happiness*

～

"I love caramel mochas… You can't take them from me.
They're my happiness."

E RICA HAD A forthright and candid demeanor. Her eyes looked at me unwaveringly. These were indications of her power, something I was to learn more about as I got to know her. I also learned about the hell in which she often found herself, and how she coped with it.

Erica suffered in her marriage, especially once she had her first child, which is when she began gaining weight. Prior to that, she had a thin, athletic build. She never worried about weight; she was active. She knew all the women in her family were over-weight and had terrible marriages, and she was never going to be that way. And yet here she was. She felt like she was wearing padding. "It's like a suit, it's not me." She described herself as "still fit, but with extra fat. *Any* fat that you can grab, that is extra —is too much."

When Erica got pregnant, she was working and going to school full-time. She quit both to focus on her baby, and after that, money became a power struggle in her relationship with her husband. He took credit cards away from her and told her that she couldn't make decisions about how to spend their money because she wasn't directly earning it.

"I wish I'd known what I was getting into. The person I thought I was with was not the person I was with," she reflects. "I feel like I got cheated."

Erica admitted that she ate when she was "upset, really angry, or really hurt."

"What's your favorite food right now?" I ask.

"Starbuck's caramel mochas," she replied, "generally sixteen-ounce. They are just delicious," she says, laughing with glee. "I look forward to them." Caramel mochas ring in at almost five hundred calories apiece. On tough days, she'd drink two a day.

She described them with such a brightness in her eye. More than joy, it was if she were talking about a great discovery, like a miner reaching a vein of a long-sought ore.

"I would leave my house just specifically to buy one, and I live twenty minutes away from the nearest Starbucks," she says with something akin to pride, then laughs. "It's dumb to place so much importance on a stupid cup of coffee."

But, as we will see, the act of getting and drinking this "stupid cup of coffee" was laced with meaning and intelligence—and vengeance too.

Erica's story would be incomplete without acknowledging the role of vengeance—a widely maligned impulse. As a dedicated believer in people's natures, I became curious about the wisdom vengeance held in Erica's responses to her situation.

People rarely consciously nurture violence. Of course, some let it guide their thoughts and actions, lavishing violence inside and out, but that is not what I mean by nurturance. My conception of nurturing vengeance is to, first and foremost, become aware of it. Then, and only then, can we make the radical step of getting to know it, tendril by tendril, agony by agony. Perhaps, rather than cutting it out like a tumor, we can determine whether it can be a seed, and identify what might sprout from it. Perhaps justice itself sprouts from the seed of vengeance. Certainly the line between the cry for justice and the shout of vengeance is blurred.

As Erica describes the pleasure of a Starbuck's mocha, I notice she's clinging to a plastic Starbuck's cup that was once filled with water. "When I get my mocha, I also get a large glass of water. It's healthy to drink lots of water." A kind of compensation, I suppose, like Erica ordering a Diet Pepsi with French fries. When we defy our inner rules, often like defying a totalitarian government, there is a cost, most of which is hidden. When most people break inner rules, we suffer an inner backlash in the form of self-loathing that follows the act. Most of us hold ourselves in contempt on a regular basis. For Erica, the water was one payment.

As she speaks, my eyes keep gravitating to her hands, curled around that plastic cup. I imagine her grasp is firm with desire, or the fear of loss.

"I keep noticing your hands wrapped around that cup. If you could show me what kind of hands those are, how would you do it?" She takes her hands off the cup.

"They are like claws," she says, as one hand curls more pronouncedly.

I'm curious to see what will happen if I try to take the coffee cup away from her. The plastic cup is too flimsy to physically fight over, so I ask her if she could notice her grasping—its nature, texture, quality, firmness, perseverance—and transfer that intention to my water bottle. She agreed to the exercise.

"I will try to pull this from you a little bit." As we look at each other, she laughs. We both know how strong and determined she is about to be.

I pull it toward me, away from her. Her muscles flex, her jaw stiffens a bit, and her eyes become even more fixed as she pulls the water bottle toward herself. She doesn't simply match my force, nor does she overpower my pull, which she can easily do. She pulls just a little more strongly than I do.

"What are your hands doing?" I ask.

"I hold onto the coffee. Not literally, but—"

I begin to pull with greater strength, Erica matching each increase. What was once a playful exchange begins to look more and more serious—as serious as her willingness to let caramel mochas cost her money, time, and weight gain.

"You can't have it," I say with one big pull.

"You can't take it from me."

"What are you grasping?"

"Happiness," she says, with a quiver in her voice. We're both startled by the quality of truth in her voice.

"Why happiness?"

"Because I don't have it," she says, and as she speaks, tears fill her eyes. "The

mocha makes me happy, in my core. Otherwise I'm impatient, frustrated." Her hands curl into claws as she describes this. "If I need it, I can go get it there."

The search for happiness is an epic, popular quest, and its trail is littered with all sorts of casualties. But Erica's vice is also a coup. She has located her happiness in one frothy drink that's only as far away as the nearest Starbucks.

After our exchange, I inquire about Erica's earlier history with dieting. I learn that she was somewhat successful in losing weight a short time ago, when her husband participated in a nutrition program that required tabulating calories during the day. He used a special computer program that translated foods into calories. Erica joined him in this process.

"It was working, but then when the class was over, we no longer had access to the computer program. We could have bought the full version of the program and continued, but I didn't."

"How come?" I ask.

"I didn't really want to lose weight," Erica says with surprising candor.

"You didn't?"

"No, why would I want to lose weight and make my husband happy? I don't do anything my husband wants, because he makes me so miserable. It would make him happy if I were thin. Why would I do that to such a horrible person?"

I found this vengeful response to be quite understandable— so raw and human. Often, in any addictive process, there is a kind of "eff you" that arises when a person uses their substance of choice against the dictates of even their own hopes and plans to desist. While this "eff you" is power that supports the substance use in unhealthy ways, it is almost always a power the person needs in order to say no to, walk away from, or resist another situation, or person, or role they are playing in life. If the vengeance is shamed, the needed underlying power will not be made available to the person, making efforts to change less sustainable.

I ask about Erica's feelings toward her marriage and husband.

"My husband is selfish and unreliable. He takes his anger out on me and assumes my motivations are not good. When I told him 'I'm going to be going to school on Tuesdays, and my mom will be here to watch the boys,' he said, 'No, you're not.' My cousin says, 'Get rid of him.'"

Maybe her cousin has the answer, but Erica will need to claim her own power and self-regard to provide herself with the way out and to pursue her happiness. We know she has this power, because it expresses itself in her ongoing Starbucks vengeance. Perhaps this energy has been turned inward, leading her to take her reaction to him out on her body.

"I do this with food too. Even housework! I don't want to clean, because I don't want him to have a nice house. I'd rather him find another nice house to be in."

The vengeful part of her is currently expressing itself via her Starbucks habit—one that ultimately undermines her happiness. She is imitating her husband in this one hurtful way. Instead of leaving her husband, she's avoiding losing weight so he won't enjoy her appearance. Instead of cleaning the house, she's keeping it messy so he won't feel comfortable and satisfied at home.

As we wrestle with the bottle, the stuff of her happiness, I suggest that I hold onto the bottle this time as if it were *my* happiness, and that she try to take it away from me. I want to explore the character and qualities within her that participated in stealing her happiness, and I want Erica to explore this thief, to "dream into it," as my teacher Arny Mindell liked to call it. I am wondering if this happiness thief is connected to the vengeance.

"This moment, this happiness, this feeling I have when I have my mocha, it's so good," I say. As I speak, I clutch the bottle and she begins to try to pull it away. "Hey, this is my happiness, why are you trying to take it from me?"

"Because I don't have it."

"I don't want you to take it from me," I respond.

"That's too bad," she says.

I hear again that clear voice of vengeance; it is a simple

equation. "If I'm not happy, I won't allow you to be happy." It is startling, but almost childlike in its reasoning and expression.

"You are not ashamed or bothered by the fact that you are taking my happiness," I continue.

"Nope," she says matter-of-factly, without any hesitation.

"I'm not happy, so you don't get to be happy," I say.

"Yep, that's it."

"What makes you so unhappy?" I ask.

"Family, my parents. They always put my sister first."

"Would it make you happy to be put first?"

"Yes, I want to be put first," she says. "I want to snap my fingers and everybody will do what I say." Putting herself first will require resisting a history of being second, or third. Much of this is also a deeply conditioned internalized sexism.

"What kind of person are you that people would do that?"

"The President. Not politically, but in a power sort of way," she replies. "It must be nice. I don't know, I never had that. I think that is being spoiled. Except I can snap my fingers and drive twenty minutes to go to Starbucks."

On one side of the fence: Erica in her current circumstances. On the other side: getting what she wants, and the label of being spoiled. On the one hand, being spoiled has a bad connotation, but on the other, is it really being spoiled to seek one's own happiness? For a woman to sometimes put herself first, ahead of her husband, children, and even parents?

She doesn't need a lot of power to get herself coffee, but she does need a lot of power to take hold of her happiness. Why? Because she deserves to be happy. But from another perspective, it is because her *desire* for happiness is powerful, so powerful that at some point she will radically change her life to get it. I think about how this challenge, if she engages with it in a muscular way, might help her to bring out, consciously, the power that is hers.

"What would you snap your fingers for and make happen right now?" I ask.

"I'd like to have my own space. It would be difficult to pack up my kids and all our stuff and go somewhere. I don't have a lot of options for that. But my husband could pack up, find an apartment, and just go. I feel like saying, 'Back off, just leave me alone for a while, I need to think.'"

When I ask her why she doesn't leave anyway, she says she doesn't think she can leave her marriage without her kids losing their father, so she can't do it yet.

Let's review this train of thought. There are two qualities embedded in Erica's caramel mocha drinking. One is her desire for happiness, the other is the power to grab it and make the changes in her life that would make her happy.

The caramel mochas are not only desirable, they not only put Erica in touch with her happiness and her desire for it, but they require something of her, a certain empowerment. She might think it's easy to go get a mocha, but to do so, she must leave the house, drive twenty minutes, spend more money than her family budget allows, gain weight, and defy her own sense of what is healthy. To Erica, caramel mochas are happiness and the way to happiness, and the way to happiness requires what she considers to be presidential-level indulgence. They allow her to claim something she never experienced before: the feeling of being spoiled, doted on, important.

In this way, the beverage connects her with her deepest desire, but it also soothes and sublimates her power and energy to grasp it and take hold of it. It is a good reminder, a placating substitute, but it doesn't show her the way. Instead, difficulty and challenge are what cause her claws to unsheathe, her self-regard and healthy selfishness to surface.

Her vengeful energy has the power, the grit, the capacity to break the rules, to grab what it wants, even if it is forbidden. To lose weight, Erica will need power, grit, and a capacity to break the rules of the status quo. And most pivotally, she'll need to change her relationship with her husband—an act that will require not only knowing what she wants, but the capacity to grab it, demand it, and make it happen despite how it looks to herself, her husband, or to others.

"If I do this more in my regular life," she says, "maybe it won't have to be narrowed down to the coffee."

"Exactly."

Erica and I subsequently developed a weight-loss program based on the insights she had during our work together. Yes, this included some additional exercise goals and an effort to be more aware of drinking caramel mochas, but the program also included getting clearer about the life changes she wanted to make, and providing her with the psychic and emotional support she needed to make those life changes.

About one year later, Erica was divorced, pursuing new career options, exercising like a bandit, and at the weight she wanted to be. A few years later, she enrolled in law school. She had snapped her fingers and grabbed her happiness. For Erica, her "hunger-thirst" for Starbucks coffee was actually a hunger for her real life, a life that would make her truly happy.

Erica's Update

Shortly before this book went to press, Erica shared a wonderful update with me. "I am an attorney now. I also got my MBA while getting my law degree, so I'm exploring the world of opportunities with my education and experience thus far. Life is pretty good!

"Working with you was instrumental in helping me realize what I was doing to hold myself back professionally and in relationships. I am very happy now with a great career, and I have someone in my life who loves and supports me in everything I am and in everything I do."

It makes me so happy to see how much power and fulfillment Erica unleashed once she stopped settling for happiness in the form of Frappuccinos.

Chapter Six

Christina: *When the Problem Behind the Problem Holds the Solution*

"Having a pizza and Coke is like a deep breath. It feels like respite, a break. I think my heart just needs a break. It just needs to be somewhere safe."

M Y WORK WITH Christina reminded me how difficult it can be for someone to have the space to attend to their own health and healing when they are partnered with someone whose addictive behaviors dominate their relationship. We ask a lot of ourselves when we try to lose weight and work out, while feeling so disconnected from our own deepest needs.

As I speak with Christina, I notice she has lost sight of the primacy of her own needs and desires. If her husband Brian isn't looking at porn or blowing money, she feels good. If he's up all night watching porn, or if she finds out he's been hoarding his purchases, she feels hurt and unsafe. Even when he is making wise choices, she lives with the fear that it could shift for the worse at any moment.

When does she have a moment to relax, take stock, and nurture her body, mind, and spirit? It's easy to get caught up in hoping a person will stop excessive behaviors related to alcohol, drugs, money, porn, and hoarding. But the most important thing for the partner is to recognize what those behaviors are doing to himself or herself.

When we begin the session, Christina tells me she has just found out that her husband is back to his old activities again. First he lied about it, then he denied that he had a problem. He also broke his promise of going to therapy.

"How do you deal with the possibility, perhaps fact, that he can't or won't stop and won't be honest?" I ask. "Let's imagine that you contact God and God says, 'He won't change.'"

"It would be a relief. I wish that the universe or God would tell me that so I could just walk away. After twenty-two years, he says, 'This is the last time. I promise this time.' And every time, I believe him."

"What part of you would always hope, would always believe?" I ask. "Tell me about her, don't put her down and tell me she's an idiot."

"I think she's the person who wants to believe that her own things that she's been putting off and not following through on have hope too," she says.

"You're saying that she needs to believe in certain things. She needs to believe, maybe not in him, but she needs to believe in herself, have hope for herself. That's very important to her. Hope is given to her and to him. And if you pull it back from him, you lose your own dreams and hopes. You don't totally believe in yourself."

"I feel like I've been able to fully show up in certain areas of my life, but there's a few areas that I've consistently been struggling with. I'm not showing up for my health, for the commitment that I want to make to feeling better in my body. It predates my relationship with my husband. My stepdad died when he was thirty-nine and I was seventeen. He was the dad who raised me."

Christina's stepfather was diabetic and took poor care of

his health. He drank and he smoked a lot. When she asked him about it, he said, "My body, my choice."

When her family found out that Christina was allergic to smoke, Christina asked her mother if she could stop smoking around her, and her mother said, "I'll stop when Sam stops."

He did stop—when he died. As Christina talks about it, she realizes that this old story of her stepfather letting his drinking and smoking hurt others and himself, leading to his death, was similar to her husband, who would not stop watching porn, spending money irresponsibly, and hoarding. Once again, "My body, my choice," even though his actions hurt their marriage, hurt Christina, and abused their household's shared finances.

Also, when Christina was a slender six years old, her mother decided they should both go on Weight Watchers. By second grade, she was throwing out her lunches at school because she was ashamed to eat in front of people.

"Yes," I say, "you're in that region of your psychological map. You're working those narratives out."

"Lately, I've been sleeping a lot. There have been so many days where I've stayed in bed until noon. That's not normal for me. And then the morning after I found out about my husband's buying, hoarding, and porn, I ordered a pizza. Granted, it had vegan cheese, but still it was pizza. And I ordered Coca Cola, which I hadn't had in probably three years."

I ask her what felt so good about the pizza and Coke.

"It's a deep breath. It's like...*ahhh*. It feels like respite, a break. I think my heart just needs a break. It feels just tired of hurting, of being on guard. It just needs to be somewhere safe. To know what's true, and to feel comforted. And feel loved, or enough."

"I see. That's important. The part of you that doesn't exercise says, 'First, I need a very safe place. Don't give me another task yet. Put me in a safe place where I'm not hurting. I can't take care of myself in a world where I'm hurting so much.'"

"And ordering that pizza felt safe, because I could eat it in private."

"That's very important. A little pizza, eaten in private, could give you a little bit of that. It's not going to create a whole safe world for you, but it's a little taste."

I ask Christina to have a little inner dialogue between two parts of herself. "It's very important to have this dialogue between the somebody who says, 'Come on, get it together, you promised to exercise, you promised to get healthy,' and the one who says, 'I need respite, I'm not in a safe place, I'm hurting, it's too hard. I understand why it's a good idea, but I'm not in an environment where I can do that.'

"If your husband were to work on his addictions, he'd have to get to know what moves him. Just like you're getting to know that you need respite, otherwise you can't resolve this issue. Saying, 'I shouldn't be this way,' is a good beginning. But then you need to discover 'What does move me? What's making me act this way?'

"What you're telling me is that the first part of your weight-loss program is to get more safety. More safety and less hurt are needed as part of your program. It's too much to expect yourself to get it together without that."

I also tell Christina that a six-year-old girl growing up with a mother needs to be told how beautiful she is, and how lovely she is, and how special she is. She doesn't need a diet. She needs to be fed affirmation. She needs to be fed safety from abuse, and lots of love. When the home doesn't feel safe, that's when people try to find the safety, to get their need met, through eating.

That six-year-old needed a safety program, not a diet program. She needed to be loved, built up, and protected.

"That's why your situation with your husband is so difficult for you. It's not because of the porn. It's not because of the lying. *It's because it hurts you.* That's the key for you. If I were you, I would not focus so much on the porn and the lying. I would say, 'The problem is not whether you're an addict or not, or whether you need therapy or not. It's not about your psychology, and your health, and whether you should go or not. The problem is that it hurts me. You're putting me in an unsafe world. That's painful for me.'"

My work with Christina brings up other, similar therapeutic experiences. I've worked with people who say variations of "I need to get my husband to stop drinking, because when he drinks, he hits me."

And I've said, "You need to get your husband to stop hitting you. I'm not saying that he shouldn't stop drinking. I'm making a distinction. Sure, let's help him not drink. But the problem is the violence."

"He's not going to stop hitting me while he's drinking."

I tell them, "You're living with a violent person first and an alcoholic second."

Christina's husband's addictions create an unsafe environment that hurts her. There's no trust, because she doesn't know how he's going to behave. It keeps her on guard. That's not a good environment.

"Yes," Christina says. "When Brian and I were talking earlier this week, I was just sobbing. I said to him, 'If you were abusing me physically, then I feel like it would be so easy for you to see how hurt I am. I wish I could just stab myself in the stomach so that you could understand how deeply it hurts me.' Not that

I would do that, but therapists have asked me to describe the hurt. I shared every detail, when I was eighteen, and then when we were married. And I guess that's why it hurts even more—because he knows how much it hurts me."

"And is that meaningful to him?" I ask her. "There's a possibility, maybe a probability, that nothing you will do will change him. There's a part of you that's hopeful and wants to believe in people and believe in yourself. That part has to believe that you're being hurt, that it's hard to take good care of yourself under those conditions."

"If he were sitting right next to you, I might say, 'Looks like he's not open to making that change. That's who you're with.' Then you'd have to respond to that—'Hmm, it's hurtful, and a hard place to take care of myself.'"

In working with people in Christina's situation, I've noticed that the addicts are not the only ones who get drunk. Not on alcohol, but on unrealistic hope. Thinking things will change when you don't have reason to believe they will change is being a little drunk. Sobriety means, "I'm not lost in believing things that are not true."

I tell her, "It's not easy to be sober that way when you love somebody and have a history. Your mother put you on a diet you didn't need when you were six, she didn't stop smoking when you were allergic to smoke, your stepfather didn't stop abusing his body, and he died when he was thirty-nine. Your husband is not making changes that would be good for you, either. You need a safer place, free from hurt, to be able to focus on yourself and to thrive. Then other things can follow from that spot."

Christina recalls the last time she felt safe. "I had some space at Christmastime, when he was gone for two weeks. Things were just so peaceful at home, and I had the organizers in, I was feeling so good, I was taking care of myself and my son, and I felt so strong."

Christina and I strategize about how she can create a safe place for herself now. She thinks about going away for a couple of days with her son.

"I asked him the day after I found out about his most recent activity if he would go stay with his parents for a little while. And he said no. If I didn't want him here, he would stay in his van. So I felt like, 'I'm going to make the father of my child sleep in his van? I know it wouldn't be me *making* him, but his van is filled to the brim with garbage, so there's only space for him to sit in it."

"He should live in there," I say. "It's not a punishment— that's where he wants to live. Your system wants to be able to tell him to go live there, but it can't yet. You don't have the full inner power to say 'Yes, that's what I want.' What if he says, 'I'll do that two days a week for the next two months? Or one day a week?' Would that be too much for you to ask?"

She isn't sure. "I don't want to shame him."

"Don't worry about that. The shame belongs to him. You should be as angry as you want, and say what you have to say. What would you say if your anger were freely speaking and you weren't afraid to be shaming?"

"I'd say he cares more about these things than he does about me."

"What would happen if you said, 'It's difficult for me to be around the lying and the pornography. It's hurtful for me, it's not making a good space for me as your person you love, as a wife, and as a mother to your son'?"

"Then he would hang his head down and put his hands over his face and say, 'I know, I know, I don't want to do this, I don't want this to be our life.' And that's when I just want to forgive him and hope that he will change."

I see that Christina and Brian have been engaging in a script of accusation, hurt, shame, and contrition—without change. I suggest that we role-play; I'll play Christina, and she'll play Brian.

I begin: "You're lying to yourself and you're lying to me. I'm not open to it. Go drink somewhere else, you're drunk. I'm not open to believing that. Don't give me your shame and your 'poor me,' I'm not feeling sorry for you."

"It's so hard when you won't believe me, when sometimes I am telling you the truth."

"Look in my eyes, Brian, I don't believe you. I do not trust you, you are not trustworthy. Don't guilt me into it, I'm not open to it. Trust is something you earn. You have eroded it, now you earn it by living differently. When I see you doing something consciously about it and getting help with it, because I see you can't do that by yourself, trust will be built slowly over time as you do that. That could mean three to six months of you doing therapy and getting help with it before I start trusting you again. That's how long it takes, that's not a long time in a twenty-two-year relationship. You want to sign up for that or do you want to make me feel bad about being tough with you? Which do you want to do? I'm giving you a choice."

"Of course I want to do that."

"Go ahead then, make the commitment. Say to me, 'Sweetheart, I'm committed to seeing the therapist for three months, once a week, and then asking you again about the trust, and then doing another three months, and asking you again, and having a six-month commitment to you, for starters.' You need to say it out loud to me. That's what's required for me to believe you, and then I have to see you do it."

"But what if it's better in two months? Am I going to have to keep paying?"

"I see. That to me says your answer is no. Your answer is either yes, and you give me those words. Anything else is a no. I heard you, you said no. There will be a point in which I am no longer here. I'm not ready to do that, I have to work that out, but I hear your answer."

"Of course, if that's what you want, I'll do it. Whatever you want."

"Then say those words to me out loud. I need to hear them. That's the first action. Anything less than that is not sufficient. I'm not going to feel guilty, I'm not going to feel bad, I'm not going to feel like I'm being hard on you. Because my hurt is so important and my ability to mother my son is so important, and you're eroding both of those. I can't stay and let that happen. I lived in a toxic environment with smoking and other things already when I grew up, I'm not willing to continue."

She is thoughtful.

"Do you think it would be fair to ask him to go for a little while?" Christina asks.

"Yes. I'd say, 'Stay wherever you want to stay. Stay in your van, stay in a motel, stay with your parents, stay on a couch, that's your decision. I'll trust that it's right for you to be wherever you are.'"

Concluding Thoughts

This session gave Christina the tools to create a safe space for herself, without privileging Brian's comfort above her own. If he were married to someone else, perhaps the porn and the buying and the hoarding wouldn't bother her. But he is married to Christina, and his behavior has been hurting Christina.

There are two parts of Christina that are in play when it comes to her health: the part that is agitating for her to make healthy decisions about food and movement, and the one that is not following through. By honoring that second part of herself, listening to it, and finding out what it needs, we have identified that what she needs is a respite, a safe place within her life to let down her guard, relax, say *ahhh*. The creation and ongoing sustainment of that space in her life is the first step on her weight-loss plan.

Twenty-two years is a long time to be in the position she's been in, but I believe in her inner strength. She's been using it to navigate her relationship with Brian, and if she continues to apply that power and strength to her own well-being, her whole life—not just her weight—will change for the better.

Chapter Seven

Kimberly: *The Mirror of Malicious Eyes*

*"I tell myself, 'Well, if you stayed on your diet like you
promised yourself a million times, you wouldn't be in
this boat. It's your own fault.' But I'm a grown-ass woman
and I can do whatever I want."*

HAVE YOU EVER mentioned to a friend or loved one that
you've been "beating yourself up" over something? The
phrase is so common that its innate violence has become muted.
The more someone knows you, the more they know your vulnerabilities. And we know our own vulnerabilities better than
anyone else. When you beat yourself up, there are no pulled
punches, no misses. Every single blow hits home with maximum
impact. Worse, there are no witnesses. No one is there to defend
you, to care for your wounds, to shed tears of compassion, to say,
"Stop, that's enough." That's how shame enters, locking your
feelings up with iron bars.

When Kimberly and I first sat down together, she told me
she had been beating herself up about her appearance since she
had her first child at age twenty. When she gained forty pounds
with that first pregnancy, she encountered body shame for the
first time.

"Forty pounds is a lot for a five-foot-two-inch person. My
doctors had told me not to gain too much weight. They kept

talking to me as if I was eating like a pig. I was really embarrassed. I remember wanting to hide, not wanting anyone to look at me."

So many women encounter doctors like this and subsequently choose not to go to doctors, even when experiencing troubling symptoms, to avoid the shaming of critical voices and cold looks when they step on the scale.

"After Valerie was born, I had to go to a wedding. I have never felt so self-conscious in my life." She laughs nervously. "I can still remember what I wore. It was a pink, old-lady blouse that covered up as much as I could cover up." At that young age, Kimberly "felt so matronly, like an old church lady. I remember wishing I had stayed home." She laughs again. "I felt really un-attractive, a very new experience for me."

When women talk about feeling unattractive, well-meaning loved ones often offer sympathy and reassurance. To truly help Kimberly, I didn't simply say, "That must feel terrible. You're beautiful!" and stop there. She is actually being beaten up. Something inside is kicking her ass. Merely offering kindness wouldn't stop the bullying, the self-abuse.

"Since then, how have you been feeling about yourself?" I ask.

"Rotten. My self-esteem is tied directly to my waistline. I've been trying to lose weight constantly for about ten years, with varying degrees of success. It was difficult to lose weight after each pregnancy, as I gained a lot of weight both times. But when you hit thirty, and then forty, and then menopause, and have a sedentary job, it's hard to keep the weight off."

The concept of self-esteem can obscure deeper issues: self-hatred, internalized self-shaming. "Wow—your self-esteem is tied *directly* to your waistline. That statement, that belief, has been etched upon the psyches of so many women."

"Excruciatingly so," she says.

"Give me a sense of how excruciating."

"I get very angry at myself for not controlling my weight. But then I think, 'Why are you so vain? You have value outside of your weight. Why are you so hung up on this?'"

She feels bad about her weight, and she feels bad about feeling bad about her weight. Women receive so many competing messages about weight loss. Even if they decide to not think about it, or aim to rise above it, they are bombarded by messages that constantly stir the debate back up inside them. An intense inner battle ensues where much of a woman's power gets siphoned off from her strength. When this is unconscious, the woman remains unaware of her power draining away, year after year, while living on this battlefield. Worse, she doesn't apply that power to other aspects of her life, like going after what brings her joy, changing relationship patterns, or applying it to her career.

"I haven't bought myself nice clothes in years because I don't want to face what size I am," Kimberly says. "I'm angry with myself for not losing weight. I care about it so much."

"Where are you," I ask, "when you feel it most intensely?"

"I beat myself up the most when I am home alone. When I'm by myself, in front of the mirror, I'm face to face with the reality that I that can't wear what I want to wear, and I get very angry. I tell myself, 'Well, if you stayed on your diet like you promised yourself a million times, you wouldn't be in this boat. It's your own fault.'"

This is a typical internalized attitude, consistent with what many people say about lots of problems. They twist the idea of self-responsibility into self-punishment and self-hate. But let's look at it more closely. A more direct version of this message is, "You're irresponsible. I have no compassion for you. I am contemptuous of you, disgusted with you. Don't come crying to me, showing your hurts and shame and feelings to me. You deserve to suffer."

It reminds me of Snow White's stepmother's magic mirror, the one that told her she was no longer the "fairest of them all." That mirror prompted the stepmother to injure Snow White. But Kimberly, like so many women, directs the violence only on herself.

Kimberly looks in the mirror and literally hears the message, "Look at you, you're fat, how are you going to go out like that? Cover yourself up." She feels terrible. That's bad enough, and then she castigates herself with "Well, it's your own fault, I have nothing but contempt for you." This completes an abusive event. It leaves a person so demoralized, shamed, and debilitated that they can't access the agency or potency to do anything. This attitude operates under the logic that people improve based on being put down, shamed, and humiliated. But this belief misses a fundamental truth: people are empowered to grow and change when they are loved, not hated.

I ask her how bad it gets.

"I had one episode in the last six months where I got very, very angry. I would never let anyone talk to me like that."

"Can you tell me what you said to yourself? Did you say it out loud?"

"I said, 'You ugly, stupid, worthless fat bitch, what is wrong with you that you can't lose a few pounds? You've been trying for so long.'"

I'm stunned to experience the vitriol and violence these words convey.

I take the role of Kimberly in the mirror. "I do try, but I seem to remain this size."

"Well, you need to try harder. There's no excuse for the way you look right now. You should be able to walk out the door ten pounds lighter, you've given yourself every opportunity, you've gone to the weight loss center."

"Kimberly, I would like to get to meet this part of you that says you are an ugly fat bitch, you are worthless. She sounds angry."

"She's furious."

"Let's hear her."

Kimberly's eyes begin to glare. I see her teeth clench before her mouth opens. She continues to viciously insult herself.

Her tirade cuts right through me as I role-play Kimberly in the mirror. I begin to cry. I can't believe someone spoke to "me" like that. We stop for a moment, breathe in recognition of the cruelty and pain that has probably never been witnessed by anyone before.

I respond, "I think you've been angry at me for long time, dear critical one. You are furious with me."

"Yes, you are a waste. You waste time, waste money, you are ugly and stupid, you don't deserve to be here. You waste opportunity. There's no excuse for it."

"You want to make me over, change me totally. How would you make me over, how would you change me?"

Kimberly stops, gets quiet, and begins to sob. "Forgiveness. Maybe I just haven't forgiven myself. I didn't know that ugliness was still there."

"What is the ugliness?"

"That voice," she says. "The depth of anger was like fire, like a flame. That type of anger is so frightening that it scares me. I can't believe it would emanate from me."

Through our joint witnessing, Kimberly begins to wake up to the abuse she lives with. It is this witnessing and recognition that brings healing to the shame that convinced her she is worthy of this cruelty.

"What happens to you when that fire and anger and assault come at you?"

"I don't know, but that kind of anger has gotten me in trouble. It hurt my marriage. I have taken such huge steps to deal with it. I thought I got rid of it."

Kimberly thought she got rid of her anger because she no longer turned it on the people around her. But it didn't go away; she just turned on herself. She didn't notice this because it was so deeply ingrained in her way of relating to herself.

"What happened after you said that to yourself?" I ask.

"I needed to soothe myself, I needed to wash my hands and face and sit down."

"You needed to soothe yourself? Where was the hurt?"

She points to her chest. "It was completely demoralizing. I felt brutalized. Like somebody knew me so well that they could go after me, with all they had, in my most vulnerable place."

"My whole personhood would be annihilated," I said.

"It felt like that was the intent. I actually felt that I was physically knocked back. There isn't anything more intimate than insulting yourself and knowing exactly where to go. It is the purest form. I've been insulted by the best, but there's no comparison. One-on-one with the woman in the mirror—she knows enough to really hurt me."

As Kimberly's compassion enters, shame's belief that she is worthy of the pain diminishes. Bringing conscious self-love where once there was unconscious hate is a life-saving response.

But what shall we do with the raw power Kimberly accesses when she's insulting herself? Will the self-love dissolve it? Sometimes this is the course of a person's unfolding, but not always. Sometimes this power needs to be owned, to become usable by the deeper life project: living an authentic life. I bring us back to her anger, allowing us to learn how it could empower her life.

"First, let's get the hurt one out of here so that she doesn't get hurt again, and then let's get to know the angry one. I sense the need to stand."

We both stand up, and she takes her glasses off.

I say, "Kimberly, you don't need therapy but this one does. How angry is she?"

"So angry that it's hard to go there. I don't like to get that angry."

"Okay, let me be the angry one." I begin. "She makes me so fucking angry, I can't stand it, I hate her—"

Kimberly grabs my hands. "You have to stop being so angry. You can't beat her up anymore. I won't let you beat her up." She holds my hands tighter and tighter.

"You won't let me do this."

"No, not again. No more," she says, with a conviction that is totally unexpected. She is determined, clear. She looks at me like there is no option. "I'm turning fifty in a few days and I'm not letting anyone knock me again. I am not going back. I'm not letting anyone treat me that way. *No*, get the fuck out." She is still grabbing me and is now pushing me backwards.

"Wow, that is awesome," I say.

"I've got my eye on you."

"You know I'll go for it."

"That's fine, I'm ready," she says.

"I haven't known you to be this clear."

"Look out, I will do what it takes. I will use everything I have, and I will enjoy it."

"Shit," I say, "I am not going to get away with this anymore. I'm sunk. I can't beat you anymore. What kind of person are you that can take me on?"

"I'm a grown-ass woman and I can do whatever I want."

"Dear grown-ass woman, how come you are here now? You seem to be very strong in my life at the moment."

"Because my knowledge has grown about my spirit, and with that knowledge comes responsibility."

"How would you deal with life differently than Kimberly the criticized one?"

"I wouldn't go backwards," she says, "My direction is right."

"Now that you have a direction, and it's a good direction, let's go for it, let's go forward. That's your message: My direction is right, don't go backwards, go forward."

Kimberly has spent the last thirty years bullying herself about her weight. As she turns fifty, she's ready to shift her power from inner debilitating criticism into a new direction, one that builds rather than destroys.

Dorito Road

Now Kimberly has seen how to transform her inner abuse into self-love and the power to follow her true path. We could have easily stopped there. This is a huge psychological step.

But these questions still remain: What is her true path? How does it feel? What does it look like? Are there any clues in her struggle with her weight that could guide her? Again, these clues are often in the hunger behind the hunger that compels eating of certain foods.

"What foods do you try to stay away from?" I ask.

"Carbs," she says. "I'm a carboholic."

"What carbs would you eat if you could eat anything?"

"Pizza, Doritos, macaroni and cheese, crackers, any kind of bread, and spaghetti."

"Let's pick one for now."

"Doritos," she says instantly.

"Let's say you had a big bowl of Doritos here."

"*Mmm*," she says intently. "Then they would get all over my hands, and they make lots of noise when you crunch them. They're salty and spicy and yummy. They're so satisfying on so many levels. I could stuff a whole bunch of them in my mouth."

"And now they are in your mouth."

"Tasty, salty, spicy, crunchy, salty, salty," she says.

"And the *mmm*, what is that like? Do you want more?"

"Always. I could eat them until I get sick. I feel content, I feel soothed, fulfilled, comforted."

Clearly Kimberly looks for *soothing* and *comfort*, but this is not all. Her *mmm* expresses something more, a fierceness that I heard in her tone. I can also tell by the way she strings these words together: *crunchy, tasty, salty, spicy*. The same inclination shows up in her psyche. She leans toward soothing, but she is also crunchy, salty, and spicy. She needs to own her crunchy, salty spiciness to free herself of Doritos, which currently is the only straightforward way she is making contact with this part of herself.

I say, "It soothes you, but not just any soothing. This is a special soothing."

"It's very tasty and yummy and rewarding. I can taste it and hear it and feel it. I want to be in a room alone with the Doritos. Don't look at me, talk to me, just leave me alone with my Doritos."

"Go ahead taste them, feel them."

"I feel really good, crunchy and tasty."

"Where is that good feeling?"

"It's like internal sunshine, I don't have to worry about anything. *Mine*, nothing else matters. There are no problems, no tomorrow, there is no yesterday, there's just right now. I am safe and warm and that's it. Nothing else matters. It's just me and my Doritos. It stops time."

"Yes, that is one of the best tastes in life," I say. "No things, no worries, nothing. Just me, myself, and I, fully satisfied. No ambition, nothing to accomplish, no achievement, no outer things. Just the present moment. I'm satisfied all by myself. Can you imagine living life from that state? 'I am a person who is wholly self-satisfied. I don't need anything from anyone or anything.'"

She is describing a state of ecstasy. Ecstasy's power is often undervalued. It's difficult for shame to exist alongside ecstasy, which provides people with a rare reprieve. Because ecstasy contains a magic that breaks people free from their usual inner, shaming litany, it has the power to heal. But if the only avenue Kimberly has for ecstasy is Doritos, she's trying to find something sacred and healing in an unhealthy form.

Kimberly's Update

Kimberly and I recently had the chance to catch up, twelve years after first working together. Her transformation and self-recovery have taken many forms: she's now an artist, a Reiki practitioner, and a counselor. She truly loves herself. In part, that came about because she decided to love her inner teenager. "She let me know that she was done being belittled, ignored, minimized. But the adult me, who has skills, decided to love the hell out of her. To accept and listen. To honor. All is welcome in this process."

The woman who used to savagely beat herself up in the mirror is unrecognizable in current Kimberly.

"Am I the weight I want to be? Not yet. Do I have the perfect partner? I have no partner. Today, I am beautiful, and brilliant, and sexy as fuck. I am heard. I hear myself. Whatever comes along next will simply be what is happening—happy, sad, scared, powerful. I am manifesting my future and enjoying my now. There is no ambivalence, only paradox. I can work with that. I am a creator. My current mantra is *I am resilient, magical love! I am resilient, magical, LOVE!*

"Do I still get scared? Oh yes. Do I still doubt? Often. But this too is welcome and has data. Healing can be so uncomfortable, especially on this planet at this time. But I heal others and my precious Gaia when I heal myself and I will not look away from my pain. At sixty-one years old, I genuinely believe that my best work lies ahead of me."

This is what *salty, tasty, crunchy,* and *spicy* looks like when it's embodied.

Chapter Eight

Isabella: *The Sweatshirt Shield*

"I needed four sweatshirts, sweatpants, and weight to feel safe. It's not because I did something wrong. It was the best thing I knew how to do to take care of myself when I was being abused."

*Trigger Warning: This chapter contains details of a traumatic, sexually violent event.

S OMETIMES SOMETHING HAPPENS to a person that triggers a traumatic response because it's similar to what happened to them long ago. All too often shame enters in the form of asking, "Why am I freaking out? What is wrong with me?" instead of "Oh, that's so much like what happened to me when I was a child. I need to be kind to myself and get support to move through it."

When a child is shamed for responding to a traumatic event—when the trauma is dismissed, denied, or blamed on the child, and trusted loved ones collude with the shamer—confusion arises in the shamed person about its ripple effect on the present, and what the truth really is. The shamed person loses faith in themselves to make sense of what happened to them and whatever happens to them in the future. That murkiness, associated with the initial shaming event, can arise again when triggering events occur, perhaps decades later, creating unconscious, undermining responses within the person that add to their consternation and self-blaming.

Isabella shared a bit about her South American background and then told me about her initial trauma which occurred when a trusted adult sexually abused her when she was fifteen. Before our work together, she had not had a loving witness of the violence inflicted on her and how it impacted her. One impact was how she lost and gained weight and how she shamed and hated her body for doing so.

"I feel disgust when I look into the mirror. I feel like I can't go outside in this body because people feel entitled to make fun of people who are not slim and fit. But it's not only about what other people think. My own feelings are bothering me a lot. I've been cooking my own meals, eating healthy food, and having three regular meals a day, but haven't lost any weight. I refuse to throw myself into some crazy diet, because it doesn't feel right. I feel that I look like a monster, and it's not a good feeling."

"Wow," I respond. "That's a strong experience. You look at your body, and this bullying, this disgust comes up, and it's strong. It's way beyond, 'Oh, you look heavy.' You see a monster. It's potent."

"Yes, it's a lot more than 'I would like to lose a few pounds here and there, and I would like to wear those jeans,' or something. It's a lot deeper and it's a lot bigger than that. When my mom sees me, she says, 'It's so nice to talk to you on the phone, because you sound so much stronger and better and optimistic. When I see you, I always feel so sad, because you look so horrible.'"

"Ouch" comes out of my mouth instantaneously in response to her mother's words.

"I agree with her," she continues. "I do look like a monster."

Isabella agrees with her mother, who calls her a monster, not only because they both think she can change her behavior and lose weight, but because they both have been conditioned to see through the same shaming eyes. She takes the monster comment in stride, registering none of the hurt the words inflict, but if she saw someone being insulted for something immutable, like their skin color, she'd be furious. People *can* change their weight, but it's much closer to the immutable category than we've been taught. Weight is a health issue, but it's also a diversity issue.

Agency around weight is so much more complicated than the endlessly proposed solution "Eat fewer calories and the pounds will come off." If a person doesn't interface with the deeper wisdom of why their body is manifesting weight, they'll usually remain at the same weight or even gain more. When Isabella's mother calls her a monster, and Isabella accepts the statement, it only reinforces the shame fortress that prevents her from mining the wisdom, the message of her spirit, crying out for what it truly needs. Isabella accepts the belief that she's culpable, and this adds to her inner confusion.

Triggered Trauma

"How many pounds are you above what you think would be right?" I ask.

"About seventy-five pounds, I guess."

"Did that weight happen gradually, or was there a period of time that it came on pretty quickly?" I ask this because a rapid weight gain can be caused by trauma, fresh or triggered.

"I had gained some weight over time, about three years ago, but I was not extremely overweight. But then I gained sixty-five pounds within a few months. It took maybe six months or so. I gained maybe three pounds a week on average before it stopped."

"What do you associate with that time?"

She pauses to think it over. "The first thing that comes to my mind is an Instagram friend, an older man. At first, and for a very long time, he was very nice and polite. He wrote to me and asked if I could tell him a little bit about where I lived, because he said that his mother's family came from South America as well. But it was all a big lie. Once I felt safe in the friendship, he turned into a pervert. It was vile. He asked me to meet him, describing explicitly sexual things he wanted to do to me. I was shocked. I blocked him on Instagram, but he somehow found my phone number and kept calling. I blocked him that way too, but he got through with text messages. Even though he was an old man now living far away, I felt so extremely fearful. I became paranoid and extremely anxious. I couldn't sleep. I went from eating healthy foods to living on hot cocoa and pasta with butter. It was a betrayal. That man had been so polite, so gentle."

"Wow. Were you aware before our discussion that your weight gain happened in response to that experience?"

"It crossed my mind, but I pushed it away. I said to myself, 'You must be mature enough to handle that stuff.' But how could he do that to me? I feel that he took advantage of our longtime online friendship."

The shame-bound mind readily dismisses self-love and proceeds with self-blame regarding the hurt and harm that others should be held accountable for.

"Yes, he took advantage of a trusting friendship built over several years. It sounds like a mirror of your early rape: that grooming friendliness, and then this. What happens to you when I say that? You don't have to agree with me, ever."

"I do agree. The same old responses came back, like sleeplessness, and locking all of my doors."

"Have you ever thought, 'Oh shit, this guy triggered my response to being abused'?"

"No, but I felt betrayed. I have thought, 'Why did I overreact to that so much?' In my country, we refer to such men as old hogs, and there are many pigs out there. If I encounter one out of the blue, I just block him."

"Yet he groomed you. He was so friendly. In your mind, you think, 'Oh, this happened a few years ago,' and then something says, 'I should be able to deal with that. It's a betrayal. There are so many hogs like that out there.' What's the voice of that dismissal? Let's say I'm you, Isabella. Let's say your job right now is to talk me out of my belief. My belief is, 'About three years ago, this old hog set me up, just like I got set up as a kid. Then he sexually assaulted me with his words. I couldn't get him out of my life. It was disgusting and abusive. It triggered my early abuse. I started eating.'

"Talk me out of thinking that. Why wouldn't I think about it that way? Because at the time, you weren't aware of how huge that first betrayal was, the first abuse. You had put a lock on that. It wasn't a part of you. It was a story, like a movie you had once seen. You didn't own the story, no one had witnessed that story. You had put it away, so it seemed unlikely that something similar could trigger such a response. What did you tell yourself, other than, 'Isabella, this makes total sense'?"

By asking Isabella these questions, I'm trying to illuminate how the triggered reaction has a distinct intelligence. Usually, people shame themselves for their triggered reactions ("I'm overreacting"), which prevents them from benefiting from the intelligence. Once in the shame fortress, as you'll see indicated by the following reply, they abandon themselves—and their own wisdom and authority.

"I told myself that I was losing my grip. I couldn't sleep at night or during the day. I'd doze off and wake up with my heart beating fast, my forehead sweating, and my hands shivering."

"You're thinking, 'I'm going crazy,' not 'This is triggering the central abuse and abandonment of my life' or 'One of my traumas has been retriggered.' Because of that shame, the denial of the actual events that happened, you just thought, 'Why am I feeling and acting this way?'"

"I just pushed it away. I thought it was too big of a reaction to the trivial online relationship."

"The betrayal by your online friend was no small thing. It would have been egregious and deeply disturbing even if you hadn't gone through the earlier trauma. Independent of your early experience, that recent betrayal is huge—and potent. That was a big, gross violation of your psyche and your body because he called and texted even after you blocked him, and that registers as danger. We live in a very violent world. Profound anxiety is a very normal reaction to that behavior."

"Yes, and then after I blocked him, he started filling up my voicemail with dirty messages."

"That's so invasive and creepy. Is it okay to repeat some of the dirty messages? I don't want the words to sit inside you alone."

The traumatized mind blurs out details. I ask her to repeat some of his messages to get to the specifics and have them witnessed, countering the dissociation that can often take over. Also, bringing the details out in the open can allow me to hold and support her powerful reactions. However, bringing these details to consciousness must be done slowly and with great care so that the person doesn't become retraumatized.

"He said, 'I'm sitting here, I'm masturbating and thinking about fucking you.' He wanted oral sex, he wanted to have other kinds of sex. I felt paranoia and huge anxiety. He said, 'I need a release here, please pick up the phone. Do this with me. I need you to call me. I need you to take me in your mouth. Let's meet, where we can fuck, and we can stay together all night.'"

"How's your anxiety doing, having said those words?"

I ask this because I wanted to see if she could handle this level of direct interaction with the triggering words and event, or if we should back off.

"I can't feel my hands."

"That's important. Let's slow down now and care for you. Put your hands together and just rub them, massage them gently. A lot of feelings want to come up."

"I can't feel my lips properly either. I'm a bit dizzy. But it's okay, I'm sitting."

"You're doing great. Thanks for telling me everything. Let's just take some breaths, just so you're here. Let's make you safer now. That was really strong, to say those things. They were absolutely gross, disgusting, ugly, mean, abusive, violent. You were abused by that man. It was a profound violation."

"Yes. He told me he had lost his wife. He had a very distinguished profile on Instagram, and people treated him very respectfully."

I can see her mind taking over to discuss the ways he fostered a feeling of safety, but I want her attention to stay with her body so we can track her trauma reactions.

"How are your hands and legs doing?"

"I can't feel my legs beneath my knees."

"Can you put your hand on the lower part of your leg, like your calf? What's it feel like there? Is it still numb? Is it tingling?"

"It's hard, it's very stiff. The muscle is tight."

I choose to help her connect with the tight muscles rather than her numbness because often a person is drawn to tight or tense muscles because they need to connect with their strength to feel more protected. However, as you will see, going in this direction was contraindicated.

"Let's now experiment with that a little bit. Make believe your hand is your calf, and you're tightening. How would your hands tighten?" While it is difficult for a person to show me the muscle in their leg, it can be useful for them to show it to me with an expression of the hand. This allows them to make more contact with their body experience and for me to bear witness to what is happening inside of them.

"Like a fist," she says.

"Feel that fist. What's the energy in that fist like?"

"It's cold. It's filled with ice."

"Cold as ice. If you can, Isabella, make some thoughts that are cold as ice. Think of a character, a person, or thoughts that are cold as ice, and the way they're said."

"My head is spinning around now."

"Okay, let's back off on that. Are your shoulders tense or relaxed?"

"They are tense and painful."

"See if they're willing to relax. Are they willing to drop down? Or are they like, 'No, I want to be like this.'"

"I can drop them down, but they are still very stiff. The stiffness goes up to my neck, to the back of my head."

There are two ways of going with trauma. One way is to go deeply into it. But if it's too much, I need to help the person find a safe place. Doing this kind of work, without attention to safety, can split a person in ways that simply retraumatizes. I could see from her spinning, an aspect of dissociation, that we needed to back up, relax, and find a safe place.

"Okay, let's try something different. Let's take our hands like this,"—I hold out my open hands—"and now we're going to breathe in and tense them. Then we'll exhale and open them up. Let's see how your body responds to that. More dizzy? Less dizzy? The same?"

"The same dizziness, but my muscles are not as tensed."

"Okay. If there's even the tiniest little thing that you and I can do to help you feel safer, I want to pursue it. Is there anything that comes to your mind?"

"No. My head is still spinning."

"Okay. You're doing great, Isabella. If Isabella's body were free, would it go under a blanket? Would it run? Would it curl up in a corner? Would it stand up and scream? What do you see? Make an image in your mind." I choose to help her step away from the strong body experiences and 'see' things in her mind's eye, giving her more distance from the event. This kind of distancing mirrors the intelligence of dissociation.

"I see that I'm curled up under a blanket in the fetal position. It feels great to do that, but also a bit awkward."

"She's under that blanket, curled up. What's happening for her under that blanket?"

"She's small, like a child, and she's very pale. She has no clothes on."

"Does that feel good to her, or would she rather have clothes on?"

"She would rather have clothes on. She uses that blanket to hide herself."

"If she could put clothes on, would she put a robe on, pajamas, sweaters, sweatshirts?"

"Yes, sweatshirts, pajamas, sweatshirts. Many different clothes. Layers. First the pajamas, and then sweatshirts and sweatpants."

"If she could put on as much as she wanted, how many sweatshirts would she put on? Just one or two?"

"Four."

"Excellent. Isabella, you're doing great. She'd put on four sweatshirts, the pajamas, and sweatpants. It's okay to be there. It's okay to put on four sweatshirts, pajamas, and sweatpants, curled up. You can do that whenever you want. It's a natural response to somebody saying words like that to you. It's a healthy response. There's nothing at all wrong with that. The only problem would be if somebody would prohibit that. A free person, a free child, does that. An unfree child may think that they're weird, and they're strange, and they shouldn't be reacting this way. A free child goes to their closet, puts on bunches of clothes and sweatshirts, curls up, gets pale, gets blurry. Somebody says to her, 'I understand. Is four sweatshirts enough, or do you want another? You can stay there as long as you want. Should I bring you tea in a little while, or not yet?'" (While I am working with Isabella via video conference and can't literally bring her tea, I am supporting her imagination of being cared for and getting to make choices about what she would need.)

"I would love some tea."

"What kind of tea would you love?"

"I would love honey and lemon."

"Okay, I'm going to get you some honey and lemon tea."

"Thank you."

"What kind of feelings are you having under that blanket, dear Isabella? Are you numb? Do you not know? You don't have to know anything."

"I'm numb, but I'm also feeling very heavy, and fatigued."

"If you were totally free, would you drift off to sleep? What would you do?"

"I would drift off to sleep. That's the best place to be."

"Isabella, I know what that's like. Sometimes I watch TV for four or five hours at a time. Sometimes I go to sleep because of that. Sometimes if I don't take care of myself, I get sick, and then I get to sleep more. It's a normal reaction. I'm so sorry, Isabella, that you had to experience that. It breaks my heart, I'm really upset about it. Somebody hurt you, and traumatized you, and scared you really badly. That's not okay."

"Thank you."

"And then your body put on sweatshirts in the form of weight. Your body said, 'I'm too small and unsafe in this body. I need four sweatshirts, sweatpants, and weight to feel safe, to feel some level of comfort. Please understand why I did that. It's not because I did something wrong. It was the best thing I knew how to do to take care of myself when I was being abused. Please be gentle with me.'"

We began this conversation with Isabella's acceptance that she was a monster. Now she's seeing how much her body's response is healthy and wise, how that's the opposite of being a monster. Reframing the way we view ourselves introduces understanding and compassion. It breaks down the shame fortress, allowing love to do its healing work.

"Yes, and the strange thing, maybe not so strange after all, is that when I think about all this, I am so much younger than my real age."

"How old are you?"

"I'm probably fourteen, fifteen."

"It makes sense, because that's when the initial trauma occurred. Dear Isabella's body, we're sorry that the world taught you to not like and be disgusted with a body that tried to protect itself. First the world mistreats you, and then treats you lousy for responding in a natural way: by eating, by gaining some more protection around you. When you were abused and violated as a young girl, you were hurt, and you responded by telling your loved ones and authority figures. Your loved ones and authority figures told you that you were disgusting for telling the truth. They said, 'What's wrong with you?' That's the world we live in. The world says, 'If someone hurts you and you tell, that's because you're a disgusting human being. If someone hurts you and you eat, to protect yourself, people say you're disgusting.'"

"You are so right. My God, how ignorant this world is."

Connecting with Her Power

As Isabella speaks about how ignorant the world is, I hear something new in her voice. She's speaking with more fierceness, even outrage in her tone. I want to support her connection with the power she couldn't access earlier.

"Say more about the world's ignorance. I want to hear."

"It's so obvious, we protect ourselves. We need comfort. When there is no one else there to comfort us, the calmness that comes from eating certain kinds of foods protects me. It calms me down, it comforts me, and then I'm shamed for it. So many people are overweight, and the world makes fun of them. They call them lazy, they call them stupid, and say 'They don't take proper care of themselves, they let themselves go. They should be ashamed of themselves. They are disgusting monsters.'"

"What would you say to them, Isabella?" As I reiterate this question, my goal is to reinforce the protective power and instinct in Isabella against her previous agreement with her mother, who called her a monster. She is becoming an advocate for others and for herself.

"I would say, 'If the world can't give it to you, try to love yourself, because you're worthy of that love. When the world laughs at you, remember that you know something that the world doesn't know or doesn't want to acknowledge. Try to stabilize your inner self. Talk about your pain, talk about your traumas. Find a witness to your abuse, if that was happening to you. Don't push yourself. Don't be too hard on yourself.'"

Her advocacy is a mixture of fierce and tender. She is reframing her vision of her weight gain and defending herself against both old inner views and the world's judging eyes.

"Isabella, what would you say to those who are cruel to larger people?"

"I would ask them, 'Why? What's inside you? What kind of pain are you carrying that gives you the right to do that to others? What are you trying to run away from? If someone is big, if someone is small, if someone looks good and someone looks bad in your eyes, it's none of your business, actually. It's none of your business. What's inside you? Stress? Pain? Frustration? Does it make you feel any better? Any prettier? Any more successful?'"

"Wow. That's powerful, Isabella. Beautiful." This is a good shift for her, to push back with critical questioning. "I hear strength in your voice, an oomph, a force, a potency. You feel that?"

"Yeah, I feel it."

"Where do you feel that in your body?"

Now that she has an inner advocate, in addition to my outer advocacy, she may be safer to enter her body experiences again. However, it still must be done with high awareness of signals that she is getting a bit overwhelmed.

"I feel it in my chest, and I feel it in my face, and my stomach as well."

"Great. In your stomach, and in your chest, and in your

face. Go ahead and play with that just for a moment. Make your face a little bit more like that. I'm asking you to do that, Isabella, because I want your body to know your strength. There are very loving and strong aspects inside you. You need your self-loving, compassionate response, 'I understand you,' as well as support and protectiveness, like 'How could people talk that way? Love yourself no matter what,' and then the strength, the indignation of the response, 'That's vulgar. I'm upset about that, angry about that. That's not okay.'"

"The world tells us to love ourselves, but it also gives us a *but*," she says. "'I love myself, *but* I'm fat. I love myself, *but* I'm not successful enough.' The message from the world is, 'If you can't be perfect, then you shouldn't love yourself.'"

"It's a nightmare condition," I say.

"Yes. I was always thinking, 'Of course, there's something wrong with me. How do they want me to act or be? Who do they want me to be in order to stop hurting me?' Because I needed them, my parents, my father. I needed a house, a home, food, shelter, some place to fall."

"Isabella, you're amazing. You are such a brave, courageous, powerful, sensitive, feeling, intelligent, compassionate, caring person, for the world and for yourself. I wish I could make a world out of bazillions of you. You are the medicine. You're the cure, not the problem. You're the solution, not the illness."

"That's very touching, David. Thank you."

"How's your body doing? How are your legs and your hands?"

"Better. I'm not numb anymore."

"How's the dizziness?"

"It's better."

"If you have a favorite sweatshirt, put it on."

"What would feel best would be to go to bed under my heavy duvet and just curl up."

"That sounds wonderful."

"I'm very grateful that I managed to connect the bad experience with my past. You helped me to see that it *was* a big thing after all."

Chapter Nine

Megan: *A Cocoon of the Right Size*

———

"I realize that hurt is the very essence of me. I don't know
who I am without that hurt."

MEGAN HAS A lot to be proud of. She has a successful human resources career involving a lot of public speaking and global travel. Her job is challenging, but she likes it that way. "I have a definite growth mindset. I like learning." She also has two children who are out of the nest and doing well. She divorced her husband about three years ago after thirty years of marriage. It was her decision, but it was still difficult.

She knows she should be concerned about her weight, especially given her health conditions: diabetes, high blood pressure, and problems with her heart. She also knows she drinks a lot (four pints of Guinness and three scotches in one sitting) and struggles with depression. She feels she "should" change her behavior around eating and drinking, but there's a big part of her that says, in her words, "You know what? Fuck it. I'm going to die one day, why do I give a shit?"

There are two territories on Megan's psychic map. One is dominated by what she internalized from her childhood: a very corrosive relationship with her mother. The other is dominated by her inner critic: a voice in her head largely internalized from her mother and ex-husband. As a child, her identity became aligned with the criticism. This leaves Megan feeling like she deserves any negative feedback, however random. When her husband criticized her, she'd accept it without any pushback.

It reminds me of the "double consciousness" W.E.B. Du Bois wrote about over a hundred years ago, although he was speaking as an African American about a racial consciousness. "It is a peculiar sensation, this double-consciousness, this sense of always looking at one's self through the eyes of others, of measuring one's soul by the tape of a world that looks on in amused contempt and pity."

How do you heal from that? One way is to become powerful enough to stand up against it. But so far Megan's been coping by drinking alcohol, because when she drinks, she suddenly likes herself and doesn't care about the criticism. Inebriation, for her, feels like a soft, safe, accepting place. As soon as her inhibitions are lowered, she eats whatever she feels like eating. Another thing she feels when she's drinking is, "I don't give a shit about anything!" This frees her from the anxiety around her family's expectations: her sister's manipulative tendencies, her mother's opinions. And most important, from her internal criticism and self-hatred about her weight.

Here's the difficulty, a difficulty that many experience: the part of her that doesn't care about anything, that is free from anxiety and criticism, is a radically different consciousness than the part of her that wants to lose weight and get healthier. Within her is a split between wanting, intellectually, to be thin and the desperate craving to feel safe and not in pain. How could the former possibly win?

She says it with more clarity than I have ever conceived: "I'm out with people, having fun, everyone likes me, I like myself. I leave the inner house of feeling like a piece of shit and go to a lovely place." The need for positive regard is stronger than any diet program's rationale, even when it comes down to life or death. When she's tried to motivate herself by thinking about staying alive for her children, that "I don't give a shit" inner consciousness is stronger. The thought that arises inside her is, "I'll just be dead one day. At least then the hurt and the heaviness I feel will be over."

What do people with addictive tendencies do? Via a substance, they practice being a certain way and having a certain feeling they don't have other times. Using the substance, they *make* an experience they want and need to be in touch with, to have an experience of themselves. Most people pathologize addictive tendencies. But we must be ever mindful that the person is hunting for an experience. Is it to go broke, run someone over, overdose? No. They are looking for something good; they are looking for home.

"It's always a question for me of sustaining. I have these incredible periods of being so incredibly clear about how I want to eat and drink. And then I can blow it within three seconds, without even thinking about it. I say to myself, 'I don't even know how that happened.'"

Megan has done a lot of inner work, but she has no idea who this other part of her is, the part that, without any awareness, in a split second, breaks the rules, jumps from her notions of clarity, and begins to eat and drink.

"I wake up every day," she says, "and I think, it's a new day. And the next thing I know, I just blew it. And how did I blow it? Where did I go, fog out, at that point?"

There's a split between the part of Megan who wants to eat and drink more mindfully and the one who goes against these goals. In other words, the one who eats and drinks is looked at as a problem, as the cause of her pain and difficulties, as worthy of punishment. While this view—that being overweight and overeating is unhealthy and problematic—appears logical and supported by the world around us, it also blinds us to the powerful needs that drive our bodies to grow bigger, and the hungers we are trying to fulfill. Worse, this view often brings shame to our struggle, adding salt, not healing, to our wounds. Once something is shamed, it eludes self-awareness; we are prohibited from getting to know what our true experience is.

Why would the psyche protect her from what's really going on there? Because what's really going on is *that* important and *that* forbidden. Because we often cannot bear the cost of awareness: experiencing the annihilating shame we have for who we are.

This "fogging out" that leads Megan to say "I don't even know what just happened" indicates that there is little relationship between the part of her who sets the weight-loss objective, and the part whose hunger and impulses prevail. There's a split between the one who says, "I'm going to eat certain things, and not others, to lose weight," and the other who says three seconds later, "I'm going to do whatever I was thinking of doing anyway."

As I work with Megan, my aim is for us to discover more about this second force inside her. Why the second? Because that first is understood, articulate, and known. The second, the one sealed in shame, is in the shadows and needs a loving witness to coax it into awareness.

I share with her that it would be good for her to get to the point where she can acknowledge her hunger, her need, her impulse to eat and drink. "Maybe I won't ever agree with you, Megan, but I better address the fact that the part of you that 'blows it' is so potent that she can turn off all your intentions with the flip of a switch, like it's nothing."

"Yes," Megan says. "It's the masked woman versus the white knight." The white knight is the one who wants to diet. And she can adopt a program with the best of intentions, but the masked woman just needs to snap her fingers and Megan will "blow it."

What is driving the masked woman? She holds the power to sabotage or to shift. But this masked woman is so used to being pathologized and shamed that she may never show up in our conversations. If we can't address her, we can't find out what inner wisdom she holds.

"It's like there's a raging battle inside my head," she says.

"Megan, I don't want you to have to be in that raging battle without the love and awareness that comes with knowing the battle is driven by your inner wisdom. You said that when you go out to a bar, people are happy to see you *as a body*, a physical human being. That's profound to me—being liked, not just for your deep intelligence, but being liked as a human being with a body. Being liked feels really good. It's more important than you may know. What's the first memory that comes up in your mind of being criticized for your body?" I ask in order to go deeper into what drives Megan's hunger to use food as a remedy.

"Really early. My mom was very critical, she still is. I would classify her as mean. For instance, I've always had long hair, and when she combed our hair in the morning, she'd get mad and hit us on the head with the comb. And she would slap me, get in my face, poke my chest.

"In a lot of ways I totally idolized my mother, because she was attractive and funny. All my friends were jealous that she was my mom. But to this day, when I hear somebody say that they love their mother, *I'm* jealous. A lot of kids got spanked in my day, but she humiliated me too. I would have preferred it if she just spanked me. She'd slap me across the face, and everyone would see the redness. It was good to go to school and leave the house, but I felt so embarrassed and ashamed. I remember going to school crying a lot, because of whatever she went off about."

"Did anyone else know what was going on?"

"My brother and sister went through it too. My father didn't get involved. I think he was as intimidated as we were. I don't think he knew what to do."

"He didn't say, 'Hey, don't take that shit out on the kids,'" or go over to you and say, 'Sweetheart, you're crying, let me hug you,' or something like that?" I asked.

"No, he sort of fogged out, or he'd leave. He'd go to work a lot." I am reminded how Megan describes herself as "fogging out" and how she works a lot, suggesting that, in a way, this is how she has learned to "father" herself.

"Work is one way of getting away. It can be a form of avoidance."

"When I was a child, we didn't have a lot of money, so if I put on weight, I'd split the seam of my shorts. That would happen a lot. And yet my mother would not either buy a larger size or repair them."

"That's an important memory. How painful. Then you had to wear ripped pants to school as a kid?"

"Yeah. As I got older, when I would find something that fit me well, I would wear it all the time. I still do it. I have an outfit that fits really well, and I wear it all the time." We can see how potent these childhood learnings, conditionings, and coping strategies can be.

"There's a part of me that feels sorry for my mother."

"Of course, I understand. And yet she passed down the

belief, 'I'm worthless,' the belief that your heart is not something to care about: 'I deserve meanness, I'm not worthy of something different.' That's the message in your father's unresponsiveness. Your father didn't respond to what your mother was doing, and your mother didn't take seriously that you'd been hurt. That very specific story inside you wants to get some healing. You don't want to be stuck there. You'd rather go someplace where you're liked, where people say, 'Oh, great to see you, nice to see you,' like your corner bar."

"And my aunt and uncle used to visit us once a year. When they did, they always commented on my weight, either saying things like, 'You lost weight,' or 'You look like you've gained weight.' My uncle would even say, 'Hey, Chunks.' Their visits would either make me feel happy or ashamed. I have a huge inner critic. I've been working on that for ten years. At least now I can catch it."

This kind of consistent critical focus on weight becomes internalized as an ever-present shaming self-consciousness, locking parts of the psyche in shame, crippling the capacity to experience wellness and esteem, empowering addictive tendencies.

"Do you remember if you gained weight in a short period of time or gradually over a long period of time?"

I ask because when weight gain occurs in short bursts, it can be easier to identify and process specific events at those times, events that can be keys to unlocking the underlying dynamics that need healing.

"There were periods where I gained more weight. One was when I went off to college for the first time. I was really miserable. I was dating a bright guy. In the beginning he was a lot of fun. Towards the end, he said, 'God, you've put on so much weight.' He was really disgusted. And we broke up after that. I lost a bunch of weight afterwards because I was pretty upset about it. And then the next time I gained more weight was when I was married to my ex-husband. He was a horrific critic. After thirty years of marriage, I just had so much of him in my head, and still do. He's incredibly smart, so a lot of his arguments were very logical, they made perfect sense."

The part of Megan who eats whatever she feels like is in a lot of pain, and is being criticized all the time.

"It's easy for you to go to that critical place. What's coming up now is how potent the critical, hurtful, abusive viewpoint is about you and your body. You can't ignore that. You will have to have a plan to deal with that.

"Megan, if the diet program is propelled in part by this disgust, by 'I don't like myself,' I don't think it's going to work. The need for love is too big, the need to be protected from abuse, which is part of the need for love, is too big. It's very significant, very potent. It's been conditioned over the years, through childhood, other experiences, and reinforced by our culture. What do you think or feel when I say that? Take your time. Your feelings are so important."

"I think that hurt is the very essence of me. I don't know who I am without that hurt. Because the hurt began with my relationship with my mother, I don't have an identity without that."

"Wow. That's profound."

"And so it's easier to put it aside, or build the cocoon to get in, or give myself a pep talk that lasts for about three seconds, and then I move on to something else. The only reason I can even talk about this stuff is because I've been a bit on autopilot all my life. At my weakest, I think, 'At least when I'm dead it will be over. The hurt, and the heaviness around the hurt, will be over.

At my strongest, I think, 'Fuck it all' to anyone who criticizes me, or ever has.'"

Megan knows she's in pain but has come to believe that the pain is the result of her size, her weight, instead of the criticism she's endured and internalized. But the criticism causes pain, and the weight follows the criticism. The dominant culture trains us to think we must lose weight to stop the criticism (and a $70 billion diet industry banks on this thinking), but for Megan, and so many, the criticism needs to be dealt with in order to address the weight issue. The weight is not the fundamental problem; eating and getting bigger is the answer to a problem. We've been trained to think that "emotional eating" is simply a form of self-comfort, instead of identifying the inner wisdom within the behavior.

"I adore my kids," Megan says, "but I can't even use them as leverage to succeed with weight loss."

"This hurt that's so core to your identity—how do you know it's there?" I ask in order to go deeper into the hurt so we can, together, bear witness to its power, enormity, and presence. If a person's hurt has never been truly witnessed, they never come to accept that it is really there.

"Because I will start to cry thinking about it, even if I can't articulate whatever it is."

"You think, 'I must be really hurting because these tears want to pour out of me.'"

"Yeah. And it's one of the reasons why I also built this cocoon a little bit more to protect myself, because, especially, there's nothing like crying at work."

"So the cocoon protects you from feeling all of that pain, from being at risk of crying in public, at work. And the other vulnerable hurting parts of you are shut off. There are parts of you that are quite alive and vibrant. And then there's another part where there's hurt, where you feel like you don't want to be alive. 'I'm happy to miss that part of my life, I don't want to hang out in an abuse scene, I can't defend myself, I'm not doing so well there.' I can see why you'd want to be dead or cocoon yourself. When you talk about cocooning yourself, do you make the connection with making a larger body or does that not occur to you?"

"Oh gosh, that never has. That's so interesting you say that."

"I've studied the issue quite a bit, and there's a very clear connection. It's far more than an interesting metaphor."

"It's really interesting that you said that, because I don't think of myself as being tightly wound in some sort of cocoon. As a matter of fact, I have this vision of a capsule with a built-in kind of bench. It doesn't have any windows. And it's blue, soft blue, fuzzy on the outside. On the inside, it's lined with long, blue, fun fur. It's big enough for me to move around in it. And it's really comfortable. It fits my size. A lot of stuff doesn't fit my size, whether it's because I'm too short or I'm too wide. It's kind of the size of an airplane bathroom. Funny that I should compare it to a plane bathroom, since I hate walking down the aisles in planes because they're so narrow, and I feel like I don't fit in the aisle or in the seat. But in that cocoon, I fit just perfectly."

"That's an amazing description. This cocoon is just the right size for you, when you fit almost nowhere else. That's what you're creating: a place where you fit just right. Soft and right. You would never want to get rid of that. You would always want to have that place to go, especially given how painful it is so often. That makes a lot of sense to me.

"If anyone says to you, 'Let's change that place that you have to go, that cocoon, to get thinner,' that's a devastating threat. It may be the only place where the essence of you, that deep hurt, can go and be relieved from the hurt. That's sacred. It's safe. But even more than that, it's a loving space because you fit perfectly, a world where you're just right the way you are."

"Yes." She is crying.

"I just feel your tears and the waters, they flow out of you. It's so hard to be in touch with the pain. It's almost like a little kid who falls and they seem fine and then the parent comes over and the kid starts crying. 'I can't cry until somebody sees it, I can't just be in this pain by myself.'"

"And my mother, my ex-husband, people don't want to see me cry. They tell me I'm too sensitive, they've shamed me."

"You didn't get what one needs, a response like, 'Oh sweetheart, you're hurting, you're showing me your hurt.' That should be met with mothering, meaning, 'When we see the hurt, how can I soothe the hurt? How can I protect you from the hurt?' The heart should be moved."

"It's the first expression of life, crying. Right out of the womb," Megan says.

"Yeah, and then somebody should take you and say, 'I got you.'"

"I got you, and how can I help your hurt?" Megan amplifies. "It's the core of life. Heartbeat, and blood, and all those autonomic things that happen in your body, like breathing."

"Yes, and the most fundamental beginning of the need for love. 'I got you.' Those two go together. It's a cry out for love, and the love should come. The need for love should never be shamed. It's the most fundamental need we have. You were a newborn. You didn't even have one percent of the responsibility to get that need met. The last time you received the soothing, the warmth, the enveloping love was in the womb, that cocoon."

"That cocoon, yes," Megan says. "There's a comfort that I can feel absolutely in my whole upper torso—the idea of being held. Skin to skin, a baby, being held at its earliest moments."

"So what I'm hearing is that you're still missing that early primal bonding, what *should* have happened. And you're manifesting that unmet need as a cocoon, as size. A place where you fit perfectly, a soft blue place where you fit. And where your tears are welcome and where the hurt knows it belongs, it can go there. You could cry until you get the need met. Maybe that's fifty more years, maybe that's five more minutes, whatever it is."

"Until I get a headache and go to sleep."

"Yes, because sleep is good, babies like to sleep. After they have a good cry, sometimes sleeping is just the right thing. Babying yourself in that way, that's what you need. It's the hunger beneath the hunger. Megan, that relationship with that hurt wants to happen. That's a very precious thing. It's happening anyway. Acknowledging it, if you can, even appreciating your body for helping you make that cocoon, will help. It's related to the flipping between the white knight and the masked woman. The comfort of the cocoon, the babying of yourself, will diminish the need for you to stanch your pain with behaviors that add up to 'blowing it.'"

"What that brings up for me is, for as much as I try to ignore my body, at the same time, I recognize it as being wiser than me, because if I pay attention, it gives me the key indicators. It's so critical to me understanding who I am."

"Yeah. It's so with us, and so rarely believed."

Concluding Thoughts

Like Isabella's experience, Megan's body's way of protecting her is to give her a cocoon in the form of a larger shape. Her desire to lose weight threatens that cocoon and has the potential to expose her tender, vulnerable, hurt self to the raw, indifferent, often hostile world. Together we discovered that she can cocoon herself in other ways—by letting herself cry and then putting herself to bed, by acknowledging that she didn't get the connection she needed as a newborn or a child, and later, when she was partnered, within her romantic relationships. My hope for Megan, as she grows into this safer and healthier understanding of her emotional needs, is that she'll integrate her desire to lose weight with her desire to cocoon in ways that don't cancel each other out; that her white knight and masked woman can join forces to champion Megan's best and highest good.

Chapter Ten

Lane: *The Power Plan*

*"There are things that I want, there are things
that I need, and I'm going to get them."*

L ANE CAME TO me as a survivor of not one but two damaging,
significant relationships: with her father and her stepfather. Her biological father was often absent and disruptive;
her stepfather was present, but physically and verbally abusive to
Lane. Lane's mother was disempowered in that she did not protect Lane or advocate for her own life direction. When we sat
down together, Lane admitted to feeling depressed and dissatisfied with her body's size. During our sessions, we began to identify the hunger behind her hunger, the message within her depression, and the path through the wounds of her childhood.

Lane describes herself as a "skinny child" until age five, when
her parents divorced. She sees herself as having weight problems
ever since.

"I lived with my mom after the divorce. My dad was only in
the picture a little. He was always unreliable, a 'grass is always
greener' type of person. In the eleven years my parents were
married, he had fifty-eight jobs! I know this because my mom's
lawyer had her count them up. He's made so many promises over

the years, but something always comes up at the last minute, and he can't follow through."

Lane's father came home one day and told his family, "I quit my job, and we're moving to California tomorrow." Because Lane's mother didn't feel like she had a say in the matter, she quit her job too and got everything packed up to move.

Some sensitive children are moved to fill the hole where a parent should have been. To Lane's psyche, the father's irresponsibility was the problem; as such, she became extremely responsible, especially for her mother.

"I am adamant about being a follow-through person, in part because I don't want to be like my dad. If I say I'm going to do something, I do it. If I'm not sure, then I don't say I'm going to do it."

Lane's mother, like many women of the time, lived unquestioningly within a patriarchal system that presented falling into step with the man of the house as the default response. If Lane's mother had been more empowered, modeling a woman's sovereignty less subject to these men's impulses, Lane would have likely taken a different path. Instead, Lane took the path of being responsible for her mother. When a child takes on a parental role, being the caretaker of their parent, their healing will later require them, as adults, to learn to follow their own life's needs and callings. When she became what her father was not, she followed in the negative space of his footsteps, and she marginalized her own need to follow herself.

Lane needs to explore who she would be without that imprint. She needs to be less responsible for others and more responsible for herself.

Eating to Fill the Hole

Why did Lane choose the moment of her parents' divorce to eat and get bigger? Perhaps, while filling the role of the unreliable father, she left a hole where her own life force had lived.

"What's driving your desire to lose weight?" I ask.

"I'd like to lose weight, but it's not about looks for me. A lot of women think they need to look like a supermodel. Not me. I like to do physical things. I like to hike. I get out of breath easily when I'm hiking or going up a hill. I have to stop halfway, or two or three times, just to make it up the hill. I'm also a certified scuba diver, and my weight really hinders me. Right now, scuba diving is not going to happen because there's no way I would be able to find a wet suit that would fit me properly. Just trying to get into it would be really hard."

"If that is what you want, what are your thoughts on why you haven't lost weight?" I ask. This is important because people always have a theory about why they don't lose weight. While they work to lose weight according to that theory, that theory is often incomplete and even part of the problem by turning the person's focus away from deeper dynamics.

"I have a family history of fairly serious depression. I think a lot of my attitudes toward food are based around that. I turn to food as something to make me feel better. My mother, father, grandmother, aunts, uncles, and cousins have all had problems with depression."

"From your viewpoint, what is depression?"

"It's a big black hole inside me that sucks everything in. It's really hard to break free of it. I use food to stave off the depression. Feeding the black hole means it's feeding on something other than me."

I am reminded of the hole left when a child fills a parental role: the hole where the self belongs.

"What do you eat when you are feeling depressed?" I ask, thinking of how she saw her depression as a beast in need of feeding.

"Usually ice cream. Peanut butter milkshakes from Dairy Queen, with extra peanut butter. I have always loved peanut butter, and you combine that with the ice cream—" She trails off dreamily.

"When you have a peanut butter milkshake, what happens to you? What happens inside your body?"

"It makes me feel relaxed and satisfied. Like a flower opening." She moves her hands and arms like a flower opening up.

It's interesting that this nature-related identification is what comes up for Lane, but not surprising, given her love of hiking and scuba diving.

"If you were this kind of flower, and you look out from the mind of that flower, the heart of that flower, talk to me, what kind of flower are you?"

"I'm peace."

"Interesting. I never saw peace with her arms up like that, opening like that." I focus on the arms because I have never seen peace expressed with arms like that. I trust that her body's intelligence is expressing something that her words are not.

"I'm reaching up into being."

"Peace, why are you here, visiting Lane?"

"It helps her be connected, to the world, to herself." She sits quietly for a long time with her arms out, just feeling. "It helps me restore connection. You can't connect with others until you connect with yourself. But more than that, even at a deeper level, my connection with the earth needs to be restored."

I never heard anyone speak so clearly about the need for their connection with the earth. Her body, the flower's message, is that the earth is her medicine.

"Why?"

"Because it was severed, damaged, hurt by the absence of my father."

"It sounds like it would be healing for you to commit to going outside, regularly, and experience the connecting."

Abuse hurts people in different ways: a hobbled sense of esteem, a broken sense of trust, heightened fear, a marred sense of beauty, a lack of belief in their intelligence, and even a profound unworthiness to exist—an almost spiritual wound. But I never heard anyone declare that their relationship with the earth had been harmed until Lane, through the intelligence of the flower, stated that she needed time alone, outside, to reconnect. It reminded me more of the intelligence and wisdom of indigenous peoples who speak more of how their connection with the earth is part of their connection with themselves.

It's amazing that drinking peanut butter milkshakes elicited this kind of insight. It did this by giving her a feeling that something inside of her was opening, like a flower, and that flower, in order to grow, sought connection with the earth it yearned to be rooted in. How beautiful that deep down she knew what had been injured and how it needed to be repaired.

Our desires have such profound and beautiful meanings inherent in them. We all own a magnificent intelligence to find our way, even in ways we would never expect. I am reminded of Jung's teaching when thinking about Lane's peanut butter milkshakes. He said that God was hidden, *deus abscondidis*, and that we wouldn't find God in churches or sacred spaces, but where we would least expect: in the dung heap. For Lane, that meant in her depression.

At Lane's second interview, she tells me, "I had one peanut butter milkshake since our last meeting, and it wasn't that good. My need has changed because I recognize what the need is for. So I now have a different way of feeding that need. I've been spending a lot of time on my back deck, by myself, with a book or not with a book, sitting or standing on my back deck, in the morning or in the night, just reveling in space. I find that it really centers me."

She did not fight the milkshake pattern; instead, she was able to integrate the impulse. Fighting with who we are only works for moments in one's life when warriorship, learning to fight, and needing to fight in life are critical attributes.

I look at Lane. She is very solid, centered, like an elder sitting before me. Her connection with the earth was giving her a connection with herself. I want to deepen her relationship with this centeredness.

"I feel an intensity in the way you are sitting," I say. "What would you say from this place, this posture?"

"I guess I would be saying, 'There are things that I want, there are things that I need, and I'm going to get them,'" Lane says. "I feel like I am going through a rebirth of Lane. For so much of my life I have put myself on the back burner. Who do I need to be for my mother, for my grandmother, for my husband, for my children, for my coworkers, for everybody else? I am finally realizing that I need to be who I need to be for me. And it's hard to fight that kind of drive within me to make other people happy."

This is part of her depression. She needs to connect with

herself. In fact, that black hole that needs to be fed was actually her own needs calling to her. In that way, the depression and the hunger both contain the same powerful intelligence. Fighting against them will only become a fight against herself, her true self.

Lane had begun to feel the call of her own needs, her own soul. Connecting with the earth connected her more to herself. Now she would need to find the power to live that connection, to live that truth. To do that, we would have to find out who stole her power. This is where her relationship with her abusive stepfather comes in.

Stealing Back Her Power

"My father was a flake, but my stepfather was even worse. I remember him calling me a stupid cunt when I was nine or ten years old. He also slapped me around, pinched me, grabbed me, shook me, and left bruises on my arms."

"Oh my God," I say, recoiling. What brutal words and hands. "It makes me teary and furious. What did your mom do?" I ask this because when the other parent doesn't take decisive action while witnessing abuse, it affirms the abuser and shames the victimized child, who internalizes the belief (often for a lifetime) that they are wrong, bad, and worthy of abusive treatment.

"At first, I would tell my mother, and she would get mad at him. He'd cry and promise he would never do it again. He would be nice for a couple of weeks, then it would go back to the way it was. A couple of times she threatened to leave." But she didn't; she was ineffectual, disempowered, a disempowerment her daughter would inherit.

"When I was about eleven or twelve years old at a picnic

with lots of people around, I got on a swing," Lane recalls. "My stepfather yelled at me from across the yard, 'Get off the swing! You are going to break it because you are the thousand-pound kid!' In front of all these people! It was very humiliating."

"That's a disgustingly mean thing to say, Lane, and more so given it was a public setting. I'm so sorry." When a person is humiliated in public, the healing problem often amplifies because it is as if the whole world were watching and either agreeing or doing nothing.

Lane managed to survive her stepfather's abuse and couldn't get out of the house and into college fast enough. She looked forward to being able to have a relationship with her mother without the burden of being under their roof. But, as we shall see, she left without the power to stand up to him—without the power to stand up to inner criticism that fashioned itself after his violence and kept her from following the dictates of her own life.

As she was leaving, he said, "Once you leave my house, you will never be welcome back again." At that point, Lane's mother decided to leave him. She asked Lane to help her move out while he was at a conference. Her mother knew there was a good chance that if he knew about it, he'd physically attack her. Lane had been ready to fill the role for years.

"My mother had to rebuild her life and not take as much crap from people."

"What did it take to do this?" I ask, knowing that Lane would also need the same capacity.

"Strength."

I notice a certain pride as she says the word—a confident, sure, articulate part of her.

"Because of my stepfather, I don't think I'm worthy of anything good, really. I hear his voice in my head, saying, 'You can't do that, you are not good enough.' That's a hard voice to kill."

"What can't you do? Give me some examples?"

"Physical things, but just a general sense of not being worthy."

"A voice says you are not worthy, you can't do things."

"You are not worthy of being loved," she says, then falls silent.

"You are in a fight with that."

"I want to kill that voice."

I want to get to know the one who says these words, and the one who is against this, and then get them to debate with each other.

"Tell me more about that voice."

"It's always been my stepfather's voice. I left his house, but I brought him with me."

Freeing oneself from the outside is a great accomplishment, but the bigger war is often within ourselves.

"Give me more of a sense of him."

"He always seemed to be angry. He was always moving, always doing more, always pushing, always poking and prodding. Nothing was ever good enough."

"If I were to talk to him, I'd say, 'I see you moving and prodding. You look dissatisfied, things aren't good enough, is that how you see them? Why not just leave things alone, sit down, take it easy?'"

Lane replies forcefully as her stepfather: "There is always something that needs to be done. The garden needs to be weeded."

"But I sense an anger or hostility."

"It needs to be done, it needs to be done right, and the only right way is my way."

"I think there are many ways, but you think there is one way, your way. Do you usually get your way?"

"Of course! I push people around until they do what I want."
In a real way, Lane needs a dose of this way of being. Instead of
accommodating others, she needs to try to get others to accommodate her—what she needs and wants.

"If someone says, 'I am going to push you around and there
is no other way to change me or communicate to me,' that creates battles."

"Yes, they see compassion as a weakness."

"There is a winner and a loser. Period. How do you deal
with that kind of situation, a pure power battle?"

"I stay away from those situations. But a lot of times I end
up forcing what I need or want down just so that I don't have to
step up and say it."

We've isolated the attacker, and Lane needs to battle with
it, wrestle with it, until she integrates some of the power to assert her desires and needs. Her belief that she must suppress this
part of herself is undermining her agency, keeping her being
responsible for others and not herself.

"He has been out of my life for seventeen years, and yet he
still plays such a damn big part in my head. Why is that? Why
is it that I can't entirely let that go?" she asks.

"One thing I know from our conversation is that the reason
it hasn't taken the next step, maybe a letting go, is that you don't
feel equipped to assert your own needs, wants, and will relative
to others. You haven't created a total freedom within yourself to
say, 'There are times when I must follow what is right for me,
regardless of what is right for others. I am going to use my
power to advocate for my own way.' Your relationship with your
stepfather is not done with you. The South American shamans
would say he is an ally, which seems counterintuitive, but I'll explain. In this belief system, an ally is a force that you meet, and

you battle with it. It could be a person, a disease, a plant. After you wrestled with it, you had a medicine that you could offer to the community. One thing that often happens is that you may walk away claiming some of the powers that the opponent had as your own. You take those powers for yourself, not to abuse others, but to serve your truth, your calling."

"In my case," Lane responds, "it is an internal struggle. This voice that I hear, that other presence in my head, is actually my own. So going to battle with it isn't really going to destroy it but make it part of me."

"Yes, as a child, you learned to go against your own needs and impulses. Instead, you learned to be there for others. Now, in a real way, you are in a battle with that conditioning. It's a shamanic challenge; you must steal the power to advocate for yourself from the perfect 'ally,' your stepfather, who pushed everyone around to get what he wanted. You need a homeopathic dose of that medicine."

We proceed by entering the battle so that Lane can make contact with this new power.

I say, "If I were this stepfatherish thing, I'd say, 'There are things I want done, and you have to do them my way, and that's the only way. Don't cross me.'"

"Part of me is actually cringing inside."

"Any particular place?"

She points to her abdomen.

"We could follow the cringing. If it were to be made manifest, what would you do?"

"I would pull in all the way."

"Go ahead, believe in your body and what it is doing."

She pulls in, crunches up with her arms around her knees.

"What is it like to do this?" I ask her.

"It feels closed. I am closing in." This is so important; Lane is being 'closed' to outer influence.

"Great, smart. Stay with that cringe, let your whole body move even further, to do even more of what it is doing. Advocate for your body and its intelligence."

In the stepfather voice, I say, "You don't seem to be open to what I'm saying."

"Why should I be open to what you are saying?" she responds, with confidence and strength.

I feel her absoluteness. In her closedness, there is a great strength that, from the outside, I can easily see in her strong back, knees, and arms that are like a carapace around her soft belly. I feel like it is already Game Over. There is not an opening for me. I hear her question as more of a declaration.

"What would you call that quality?" I ask.

"I've gone from cringing to strength," Lane says. "I really feel strong right now. It's like I've pulled in, put up my defenses, and I'm ready to go. Ready to fight."

"I feel it. If something says, 'You're not worthy of doing certain things, you should focus on other people,' what would you say?" I ask.

"Bullshit."

"But aren't other people important?"

"Yes, but if you are not strong, if you are not well, then how can you give?" she responds.

"Should you focus almost exclusively on your own needs and wants?"

"No, I have children."

"How do you know whether to fight for your own needs or not?"

"I don't know, I am still learning that." Lane smiles. "But I feel the readiness to fight."

Concluding Thoughts

Lane's two fathers violated her: one with neglect and irresponsibility, the other with direct aggression and abuse. Without a mother to stand up to these forces, to model self-responsibility and empowerment, Lane got sucked into the role of being responsible and protective. Not only is this role unhealthy for the child, it can lead the child, as it did for Lane, to abdicating responsibility for their own needs, impulses, and path.

Lane's growth required that she deal with the impact of these two fathers—first, by connecting with her own needs and impulses, and second, by connecting with the power to stand for those needs and impulses.

What did I learn about Lane's weight issues? Lane had a hole inside of her, a hole that prompted a hunger to fill it. She called this her depression, something she fought against. This hole was not a destructive pit to avoid but a powerful hunger to become her true self. As she connected more to her true self, which manifested in our session as her identifying as a flower hungry for connection to the earth and nurture from the sun, the hunger began to subside.

But connecting to her self in nature was the first of two important and interdependent steps. She also needed to claim the power to advocate for that self against the pull to be there for others. The power struggle with her internalized stepfather was the training ground for developing that power. This is a rare step for many, as most of us want to be nothing like a person who abused us. Of course, we needn't use the power to abuse others, but if we turn away from those powers in total, it may cripple us from claiming the powers we need to support our own life project. Lane and I took a first step when we consciously engaged in that struggle. She then experienced how that power would serve her.

Chapter Eleven

Jasmine: *You Don't Hurt Things that Are Beautiful*

"As I got older, I noticed thin white women, their body types. I will never be a size four. However, some part of me absolutely wishes I could be. Does that mean I want to be like a white woman? Isn't that self-hating?"

JASMINE IS A forty-one-year-old woman who works at a company where she is one of only three African American women out of 150 employees. She often has trouble breathing because of allergies and anxiety. She describes the sensation of an anvil on her chest, keeping her lungs from expanding. Sometimes she takes medication, but it can exacerbate her symptoms and make her more anxious.

(As I write this chapter years later, I wonder whether Jasmine knew that African American women were twenty percent more likely to have asthma than non-Hispanic whites and almost three times more likely to die from it. This is important because symptoms of all kinds, including emotional and physical, can be race related, meaning they can be caused by or amplified by the racism that exists in the history and culture of the U.S. and many of its organizations. Seeing her allergies and anxiety as only an individual problem marginalizes racism's impact, reinforcing the idea that she has something wrong with her instead of including the understanding that there is also something wrong with the world she lives in. The belief that "something is wrong with me as an individual, as a person," breeds shame.)

Jasmine agreed to participate in my research because she wasn't comfortable at her current weight. Jasmine's body journey reflects not just her genes and eating habits, but the effects of racism: being deprived of the power and control that privileged white people take for granted.

At the beginning of our session, she tells me about a recent dream. She was trying to get away from the police who were chasing her. Eventually she parked her car, and a friend said, "Here is a car for you." It was a beautiful, colorful convertible Cadillac. She wanted to take it but thought if she did, she would certainly get caught because it was so flashy. She thought, "I should drive a PT Cruiser instead," although that car didn't appeal to her.

This dream turned out to be quite prescient, as dreams often are. It showed her being chased by something and that she had two alternative modes of responding: showing up dazzling and flashy (something we would learn more about) or blending in, being less visible. This is a decision almost all marginalized groups of people face: *How much will I assimilate, accommodate, so I, as an innocent person, don't "get caught"?* When I say "get caught," I mean anything from getting dirty looks from a stranger who thinks they shouldn't exist, let alone be flamboyant, to getting pulled over and subsequently shot by a police officer while unarmed and compliant.

And, what will be the cost to my culture, soul, and body of this assimilation?

"You can put yourself in a smaller, less flashy car in life," she says, "but can you get away with that? I don't think it will feel very good. But, on the other hand, if you take the Caddy, you'll get caught."

"I'm hearing that race and racism is part of talking about weight for you."

"Absolutely," Jasmine says.

We then spend time talking about African American women and men who are powerful, who are *out*: resplendent, expressive people like Maya Angelou and Cornel West. Jasmine doesn't feel comfortable being that way at this point.

We decide to consciously investigate how her struggle with her size and weight is a manifestation of this central dilemma as a black woman. Is there a key to becoming smaller, or is she actually hungry for a deeper understanding of her body size and shape?

Jasmine's Personal History

When Jasmine was twelve, her older sister died. For years she told people she was an only child, trying to act like her sister was never there.

"She killed herself. She was very thin, a size six. I remember thinking, 'Wow, I can't even fit into her clothes,' when she was ten years older."

The issue of body size, body shame, was present even then.

Jasmine took a deep breath. "I feel a deep anvil in my chest as I speak about this."

The intimate connection between the body's symptoms and our emotional life is rarely considered. This anvil, easy to label as a manifestation of a physical illness like allergies or lung problems, is clearly also related to an emotional experience. It's not that our emotions *cause* our physical symptoms, but they *mirror* each other. The body and mind are not separate; they often speak together.

Jasmine's perspective about her body size was influenced by both her family culture and the dominant white culture, which differed.

"Inside the house, we never worried about weight or talked about size in my household. My mom believed in meals, not snacks. In the morning, we had eggs, toast, cream of wheat. I filled up on food, not snacks and desserts. Outside the house, it was a different story. In second grade I remember a girl who was teased on the playground for being fat. The boys called her Fatty, Porky. I felt bad for her, noticed they were hurting her feelings."

(I didn't ask about the race of the girl or boys until later, but, dear reader, perhaps you have a guess.)

"And then I thought, 'What about me? Maybe I'm fat.' I was a solid kid, not really flabby, just a healthy kid. I didn't think about it a lot or come to a conclusion about my weight. But the seed was planted."

Jasmine, like so many women I interviewed, had a similar early story where the seed of body hatred and shame was planted.

It would be easy for many not to see the racial dynamics intricately woven into this dis-ease. It would be easy for many diet programs to treat her as an individual who needs more discipline or healthy eating habits, dismissing the fact that Jasmine has no interest in dieting, and that there was no body shame within the culture of her black family. Any weight-loss program that doesn't see the racial implications would bring shame to Jasmine by neglecting to identify racism's impact on her image of herself.

For example, let's say Jasmine, or another woman of color,

goes to a weight-loss coach and says, "I want to lose weight." If the coach doesn't ask why and come to understand the racist eyes that see her as fat, as too big, then the coach will buy into racism's hurtful eye. This can amplify the internalized racism that some women of color experience regarding their bodies when the white cult of thinness is imposed on women of color. Failure to bear witness to racism's effect on black women's body weight and body image hardens shame through its complicity with white standards of beauty.

The Double Bind: An Ethical Dilemma

Our conversation continues by exploring more of the double standard she was subject to.

"As I got older, I noticed thin white women, their body types. I will never be a size four. However, some part of me absolutely wishes I could be. Does that mean I want to be like a white woman? Isn't that self-hating? That's really disloyal."

I recalled Karen Pyke's understanding of this dynamic in her 2010 *Sociological Perspectives* article, "What Is Internalized Racial Oppression and Why Don't We Study It? Acknowledging Racism's Hidden Injuries," when she wrote, "The imposition of White beauty standards can cause some racial minorities to feel unattractive and to desire more White-like features."

I ask Jasmine if she feels comfortable role-playing to investigate this double bind of either feeling discomfort for having a large black body or feeling disloyal for wanting a thin white body. She agrees, and I begin, saying, "'I wish I looked like the thinner white girls and women.' What would you say to me?"

"You can't think that way, that's so unhealthy," she says. "You have to find a way to feel that you are beautiful."

"I can't do that. I absorbed this belief my whole life. I don't know how to do that."

"I don't either, but we have to find a way. I tell people that I weigh between 180 and 190, but I actually weigh 225. If I could get down to a size ten, that would be terrific. Size six would be even better. Size ten is okay, but it's not my ideal."

Neither Jasmine nor I know the way out of the harm this racialized view creates as she begins to reveal the shame that leads her to hide her true weight.

I remind her of her earlier statement. "Maybe being a size six is deadly. The story you told me of your sister shows the potency of that particular size."

Jasmine wouldn't identify as suicidal, nor would she see herself as following in her sister's footsteps. But there are other ways of killing oneself a little bit every day, by covering up, blending in, and not showing up as we truly are. Externally, racism kills people directly through bodily violence and with its steady drip of hatred and fear-inducement. Racism also kills from the inside when it's been internalized.

"Exactly," she says, "and I am starting to see how size can be a life-and-death issue, given how many people die from eating disorders."

Jasmine's awareness is mirrored in how this understanding has been growing in recent years as more research emerges about eating disorders among black women who were earlier underrepresented in studies, which infuriatingly led to assumptions that they did not suffer from bulimia and anorexia. Research is now educating us about how acknowledging the stress of both current-day racism and generational trauma is critical to truly understanding the role of eating disorders in black women's lives.

"Right. When you say you are thirty pounds lighter, that's

a little death of that unaccounted-for part of yourself. It's an accommodation to a norm and culture that is not truly your own. What does it mean to be a size six?"

"Thin, white—it's the way it's supposed to be. It's control, not only over certain people. It's control in that things come to you more easily. You don't have to work as hard. It's lighter, not as heavy. I have to suffer indignities, small ones, all the time. For example, I got an email at work that was addressed to another woman—another black woman. There are only three of us out of 150 people. It's like, 'You motherfucker.' I always have to hold myself in check."

"So that your job is not threatened, because it could be deadly to your status at that company. So you didn't say anything, even something far less inflammatory. You didn't take the Cadillac."

"Exactly, I took the PT Cruiser."

When Jasmine chooses the PT Cruiser instead of the Cadillac, even in her own mind, she's stifling and suffocating the part of herself that identifies with the Caddy, out of fear of what would happen to her—from discrimination, to ridicule, to harassment, to death—if she went ahead and embodied her innate sparkle.

It's not surprising that Jasmine feels drawn to being thin and white, because they are allowed to be fully out—visible, supported, and given a lot of leeway to be flamboyant and fierce.

"Can I ask about the race of the girl in your second-grade story?"

"She was black."

"And the boys?"

"Oh my God, they were white. I didn't even notice that until now. I can't believe it," Jasmine says.

This is part of the shame induced by a racist culture that

encourages, even dictates, that race is not a factor, that color ought not be noticed. But this blinding is internalized, making the world colorless, obscuring the dynamics of racism from people of color.

What's the impact? People aim to identify their own limits, errors, frailties, and pathologies rather than seeing a racist culture's impact. In effect, they blame the victim: themselves.

"I get the appeal of being thin and white," I say. "Control, ease, power, freedom. That's a very compelling offer. Who wouldn't be seduced?"

"Right?" Jasmine says. "And you'll be safer too. There's a sense of being protected. You don't hurt things that are beautiful in your environment. Men protect you! You can even use your power for good, to do things. It's an all-around good thing—it's a panacea!"

You don't hurt things that are beautiful.
This is such a powerful theme.

Although the reality is far from unblemished—men rape, beat up, and murder beautiful, thin white women every day—the belief has power, not only for women who are, relatively speaking, more protected, but also for women who feel like they don't fit into a protected category.

"Wow, it's like being thin and white is the answer to life," I say.

"Absolutely," she says, comfortable and clear.

"Do you actually want life to be easier, safer?" I ask.

"Yes," Jasmine says, "because when your life is easier, happier, you put beautiful things into the world. You get all the other things out of the way." As she says this, I am seeing the colorful

Cadillac of her dreams and wondering what form the beautiful things in her would take.

"What could you do if you had this safety and privilege?" I ask.

"I'd be kinder and easier on myself. I wouldn't struggle so much with feelings of worry about what's going to happen next. I would really be able to help people who need help."

"I see. First it would ease your anxiety, and then it would help your gifts come out. What would come out more?"

"Love, kindness. There's a lot of love in me." Her eyes fill with tears. "Wow, that's emotional for me. I think it doesn't come out very often. I worry that it will be damaged. My love wants to come out, but it's not always safe."

"Ah, so the Cadillac, the beauty that is in you, is your love. Wow. But you're choosing the PT Cruiser instead, to lay low."

Working Somatically: Anxiety's Anvil

As our conversation continues, Jasmine puts her hands on her chest. "I want that anvil off my chest."

"Can I put my hand on your hands?" I ask. "If so, I am going to be a little anvil-like." I ask so that she feels safer with my touch, but I still must listen carefully to see if she is hesitant, because not everyone can say no easily.

"Yes, my heart wants to stop the pushing," Jasmine says, as if her heart were pushing back against the pressure.

"You can push my hand back, with all your intention."

She takes a deep breath, pushing my hand out by expanding her lungs. I know we are in an important place because she said earlier that she had breathing problems. I now see that pushing back against the anvil is a kind of medicine for that problem.

Wanting her to be less vulnerable than having my hands close to her chest, and wanting her to access more of her power, I suggest we stand up, face each other, and have her hands push against mine. "Let your hands push like they are part of your chest, like they are part of your breastplate."

She gives a good push, saying, "I can't totally let it go, but I feel calmer now. I got that out."

"So this is part of what your anxiety is about. An anvil is on your chest and your heart is pushing back, making you calmer."

"I went through a long period where I didn't really feel safe to push back. But now I'm living again."

Concluding Thoughts

Jasmine came to me hoping to find ways to lose weight. Was it because of health reasons? No. Was it because she wanted to be more beautiful or attractive? Not really, because as we learned, she didn't feel unattractive in the world of her black family, only in the white world.

Why did she feel moved to make efforts to lose weight? Jasmine wanted the protection, support, and freedom that went along with what it meant to be thin and white.

And what is the benefit she imagines getting if she lives a life with the privilege and advantages of being thin and white? She gets to bring out her deepest self, her deepest gift: her love.

How will Jasmine get there? How will she achieve this end if she doesn't do it by losing weight, which holds no guarantees of getting her there? She needs to push against the system that suppresses her, inside and out, so she can move, love, and create in the world like the resplendent person she really is.

Chapter Twelve

Francesca: *Breaking Out of Smallness*

"I'm a huge thing. If you only give me a small task, I will create big difficulties to satisfy my huge hunger."

F RANCESCA HAS BEEN incarcerated more than once for drug-related transgressions. Most recently, she spent two years in the penitentiary for drug possession. Had she shown up for her court date, she might have gotten a lighter sentence. This was not the first time she didn't show up to court or violated her parole.

"Why didn't you show up to your court dates?" I ask.

"I would never go to court unless they caught me and dragged me in. Why would anyone go to court—so you can turn yourself in and get locked up in prison for two years? If I knew I was going to prison, I would act like I was drawing a gun on the cops so that they would kill me."

Francesca is not in prison now, but as you'll see, she experiences normal life as a kind of prison. She's in school, but doesn't want to have to work at the same time because she fears that her grades would suffer. She has hepatitis C. She definitely doesn't want a normal job. She identifies as a breakout artist. Using drugs has given her an instant way to break out of her normal life.

Francesca has been out of prison for ten years, but before

that, she was often in jail. She went through a period where she would violate parole, not go to court, and get thrown in jail. Francesca says she was a very free person, but her desire to be free caused her to buck the system, and she paid for it with more time behind bars. One could say she dreams of being in prison so she can contact her impulse to break out. This unconscious pattern can also be found in many dieters. They dream of feeling better about themselves by losing weight and then break out of a weight-loss plan based on self-criticism and body shame. Freedom, however unconscious, is a very powerful force.

Francesca was always a free spirit; it was never easy to contain her or lock up her in any way. In fact, when I ask her about her early memories, she begins talking about experiences she had at just a few weeks old. (The first person I ever heard recall stories from this age.)

"I was in my crib. I was born with two teeth. When I was two weeks old, one of the teeth got stuck in a loosely woven blanket. I had been crying and flailing, and my tooth got caught in the blanket. I yanked the blanket and ripped it out. It startled me."

Even then she couldn't be held back, ripping out a tooth to set herself free.

By the time Francesca was five years old, her father was no longer around. She had four brothers and sisters. "We were cooking our own meals and on our own. Mom would work at night, we would get up for school on our own, we would come home, and she would already have gone to work. By the time she came home, we were in bed."

Drugs were Francesca's way out. At seven years of age she smoked her first joint. By thirteen she was injecting methamphetamines.

"For the most part, methamphetamines raised me."

Francesca never had it easy. She was always up against difficult odds and overwhelming circumstances, but she also survived and fought for her freedom. In some ways she was equal to any foe, any hardship. Some children soften, wither, and withdraw—not Francesca. She grew strong, fierce, and determined —a freedom fighter from the get-go.

"The survival instinct in me must be huge. Even when I don't want to fight, I do. When I was in prison, I was the smallest girl, but for some reason, even the biggest, toughest women were afraid of me. Later I set myself up with a guy who would abuse me, try to kill me."

The Smallest Kid

Francesca was one of the smallest women who participated in my study. Unlike other women who reported having struggles with weight as children, Francesca was always quite small.

When I ask her about the first time she became aware of her weight, she says, "When I started school at around age five, I remember being smaller than most of the kids. In seventh grade, the kids were wearing size one or size two, but I was still wearing little kids' clothes. The other kids' clothes were more adult-like, not mine." When I tell Francesca that by fourth grade most girls are struggling with seeing themselves as too heavy, she is shocked; that wasn't her experience. Instead, Francesca wanted to be bigger, not smaller. "When I was a kid, I felt small, like I couldn't protect myself. I was picked on, chased by kids. They said I was different than them."

Yes, some people eat to get bigger or, more accurately, to get in touch with their bigness!

"What could you have done if you were bigger?" I ask.

"Beat 'em up." She laughs. "I always was picked on by the biggest, I was always the smallest. My dad and mom, drunk and fist-fighting, my older sisters and brothers picking on the younger ones. I guess this bigger-smaller dynamic was always around, now that I think of it. When I went to prison the last time, I was the lead baker, and I put on lots of weight."

Big forces stalked Francesca, whether they were older siblings, terrible childhood conditions, drugs, abusive men, or prison. One of my teachers once told me that big gifts dream of big difficulties. He was suggesting that we are not only victims of the forces against us; the great forces in us almost invite great, equal, and opposite forces against us. This was certainly true for Francesca. The question is: How will Francesca connect with, embrace, and own how big, how powerful, a person she actually is?

Francesca's Experience of Her Body

"How do you experience your body nowadays?" I ask.

"I feel obese. I get hungry and I eat, which is all the time. I know I should be exercising and not eating sweets."

"How do you know you're obese?" I ask. While this may seem like a senseless question, shame targets specific areas of our bodies—our arms, cheeks, thighs, or bellies. To get in touch with the body battle she was engaged in, we needed to find out specifically where the shame lands.

"Not so much from the outside. I look in the mirror and see disgusting fat on my legs, on my stomach, my arms, all over."

To amplify her view of herself, I ask her to make believe that I am that "Francesca" in the mirror.

"Talk to me, tell me what you see," I say.

"I would say, 'You are disgusting, you need to lose weight, it's gross. Look at your arms. What can I wear today to cover you up?"

"What do you mean, I'm gross?" I say.

"You are fat and flabby and disgusting." We have achieved the necessary specificity; the contempt in her voice is real.

"What's so good about no fat? You are disgusted with me."

"Yes, I don't want anyone seeing me with my clothes off."

While Francesca once fought great forces on the outside—siblings, other children, horrific childhood conditions, drugs, fellow inmates, abusive men—she now fights different foes, but similar powers, on the inside. Her body and her view of her body provides her a battleground, much like her outer struggles did.

Like many women, Francesca is a powerful person who is not free to express such power. And so her power is split off, showing up in less conscious, less deliberate, and some would say, less healthy ways. For some women, this less conscious power manifests in potent self-criticism and powerful inner battles with that criticism, especially with regard to their body.

We can now see the critical dynamics working against Francesca losing weight. First, Francesca's impulse to be bigger is based on the need to protect and defend herself—to love herself. Second, she makes contact with her power by battling great forces. She has found a battle that the culture readily provides—a woman battling with her body image.

To further unfold the power pent up in her weight struggle, I ask Francesca more about her experience of being criticized: looking in the mirror and seeing fat and being disgusted.

"How do you feel when you are criticized?" I ask.

"I feel shame, self-loathing. I have had those feelings my whole life."

"Where are those feelings the strongest?" Because her struggle is in her body, I want a response from her body.

"Stomach, head, and heart."

"Help me feel the way you feel physically."

"Tightness, anxiety, clenching, tension." She clenched her hands.

I see that her hands are making a grabbing motion as she speaks and ask her to grab my arm the way her hands were grabbing and clenching before.

"Really do it?" she asks, and laughs as if I were crazy, knowing how strong she is.

"Do it twenty percent," I say, remembering that she may look small but is actually quite big.

She starts, then stops. She looks disoriented. She starts again, and begins to cry.

"I've been on this kick lately about how I feel about myself, and how it never seems to go away. I can't make it go away."

This has always been true for Francesca. There is so much feeling, energy, power, and frustration wrapped in her experience, and now, her experience has been exposed, before us both.

"You brought this memory back to me of when I was two. I had this little stuffed doggie, I loved that dog. I would get so angry, I would squeeze it and grab it." She wringed her hands as if she were grabbing and twisting a pillow.

"It's inside," I say.

"Yes, it's inside. It's bad."

I grab a pillow, growl, and twist and squeeze it.

"Yes, rip it apart," she says, and smiles and laughs nervously.

"Let your mind become the mind that would do that," I suggest.

"I don't know that I want you to see me like this." Now we

are close to the root of her struggle. She not only doesn't want people to see her as fat, she doesn't want people to see her as fierce and powerful as she actually is. Until she can become unashamed, unafraid, of her own power, she is likely to gain weight to make herself bigger. The body is miraculous in this way, carrying the issues we can't resolve in size, shape, and symptoms.

I encourage her further, and she begins to growl and twist the pillow.

"Yeah, but louder. The loudest and most wrenching noises anyone could ever make."

She's really getting into it now.

"A few men have said that they were intimidated by me. As if I'm like Bigfoot, the Abominable Snowman." She stretches out her arms. "Huge, almost godlike, it's so enormous."

One can't easily contain Bigfoot, even by trying to convince her to eat more healthfully. Before Bigfoot can go on a diet, she must realize that she is Bigfoot.

"Sense that in yourself. Let go of your normal reality, your usual sense of yourself."

In a real way I am asking Francesca to break out of herself—her smaller, less empowered self. I am hoping she will connect with her power, identify with it, own it, become it for a moment. I hope she will enjoy it, befriend it, so she will no longer turn against it, so she can live out loud. So she can love who she really is—a powerful woman.

"I am afraid of it. It's scary. I want to go run and hide. It's like when I was a little girl. I had this dream that there was this thing that would chase my entire family. In the dream, it knows where we are, and my dad stands up and tries to protect us."

That thing in Francesca's dream is her—her power, the thing her family was rightly frightened of as she broke out and confronted their denial, patterns, and abuse. People often find themselves running from something in a dream: a mist, a monster, a parent, a faceless creature, evil, a tiger. But what if we don't run from it? What if we face it? We may find out that the monster is our power—a power that family and culture has taught us to be afraid of. This is where we go next.

"Sense your Bigfoot self again, feel like it, be it."

"Nobody could hurt me, they would be afraid of me. Nothing could hurt me. Nothing. Just the shell of it could stop a nuclear bomb."

"Nothing can hurt you, Francesca, nothing," I say.

She begins to cry. "I need to sit down."

Francesca needed some of this protection in her life as she was growing up, getting beaten up, abused, using drugs, being in prison, not having the protection of her parents. But as I got to know Francesca, I believed she not only needed this as a younger person, but she would still need it. Maybe she would have to face down her addiction again, or fall prey to it and the dangers of that lifestyle. Maybe she would take on big tasks worthy of her power or step out of conventional sexist roles in relationship.

She begins to tell me about a story she heard of the Loch Ness monster. "A boy found it as an egg," she recounted, "and it grew to be this huge Loch Ness monster. The little boy would go back and see it, the monster would take him swimming. The army came to kill it. They shot at it, but nothing could hurt it."

An army couldn't kill it, but it befriended a little boy. Francesca is telling me her own story, including the story of her drug use, and later her weight gain—how it befriended her, helped her through, from a very young age. How it couldn't be killed even under enormous attack. That Francesca has been off drugs for years means she must have found some way of befriending this monster along the way.

"I used to think that God sent the drugs to me because it took the pain away. I don't think most people would be able to survive what I've been through."

"It can be a friend that can sometimes do more than take pain away," I say, thinking that drugs not only took her pain away, but was her way of accessing the monster.

"Yes, it is capable of murder sometimes," she says. "I'm seriously afraid of that part of it. It is related to that part of me that doesn't want to be hurt. When I get hurt, it grows so huge and so destructive. In a sick way, I kind of love it too. But it's not healthy."

"Not healthy in some ways, and protective and empowering in other ways."

I want to continue unfolding the relationship between Francesca and the monster. If she turns against this monster or tries to get rid of it, even by dieting, it won't work. The monster is an ally, not an enemy, in all major areas of her life.

A Dialogue with a Monster

I decide to play the role of Francesca and ask her to play the monster.

"I needed you, you were there for me, you protected me," I say. "You were always there for me, nobody else was. How come you were always there for me?"

"Because they were always hurting you," she says.

"How come there for me, why not there for someone else?"

"Because I love you." She begins to sob. "Nobody else does."

"You love me?" I ask, as if I didn't know that, wasn't sure of that.

"Yes," she cries even harder, "it's kind of an intense thing."

"You're full of love."

"I think only for you."

"Sorry that I think of you as a big nasty monster," I say. "I have a big, huge friend who is always there for me, who loves me."

Francesca cries and cries and cries. We hit pay dirt. What she learned was unhealthy, what she learned to be afraid of, what she learned to suppress was actually loving herself.

"Why doesn't it crush the addiction?" she asks impatiently.

"I'm a huge thing. If you only give me a small task, I will create big difficulties to satisfy my huge hunger. I'm not going to crush the addiction until something big enough, as big as the addiction, as huge and as wrenching, fills your life. When that happens, I'll crush the addiction like a—"

"Like a bug," she says, and laughs with recognition.

"I need something big, I want to rip teeth out," I say, remembering her early memory.

"That's right, exactly. That must be why prison was such a huge thing for me."

Let Me Eat Cheesecake or Let Me Die!

All diet plans and weight struggles set up a wrestling match with eating: what to eat, when to eat, how much to eat, and why you eat. Within these deep longings for foods, people are reaching for some profound state. In short, we are all hungry for who we are.

Francesca longs for fruit cheesecake. "I make the best cheesecake. But I have to make at least two, because if I don't get a whole cheesecake for myself, then I feel robbed. It has to have a graham cracker crust with real butter." She is a connoisseur; she knows, down to the detail, what she wants, what she likes, what she craves. Someone might say she craves sweets, but then why the real butter, why the fruit, why the graham cracker crust? No, Francesca, like others, has a desire at once quite specific while also quite deep and profound.

"What's it like to eat a cheesecake?" I ask.

"It's like an orgasm. Mmm, it's love."

"Here, take a bite." I motion to her like I am giving her a piece of cheesecake. Francesca sighs as if delighted.

"What happens to you?"

"I feel loved, I am reminded of the monster. It's relaxing, it's acceptance, it's like finally coming home. Home is such a big thing for me."

Because home is a place of safety, a place where she has a monster to protect her, which she didn't have—she looked for it in drugs, and in a sense, found a version there—and which the monster has tried to help her create.

"Tell me more about home." Now that Francesca has made a deeper relationship with her power, I want to help her think about a life beyond wrestling with food, drugs, and prison, not by trying to get her to go on a diet, but by integrating her power and being fueled by a deeper self-love.

"When I was fifteen, I overdosed. I left my body. It was so awesome—I was this gray mass. My friends were there, screaming my name. I was weightless, I was swimming and floating and giggling and doing these weird twirls. That's home." Many people would try to dissuade her from thinking this way, but that only shames a person for having and desiring a profound spiritual experience. To help a person not use dangerous drugs to find this state, the state, not the drugs, must be valued.

"Let's go back to that state. What kind of life would you create?"

"Anything I wanted. I was myself, but I was everything, or at least I was a vital part of everything. But something made me go back, and it was so disappointing. It made me so angry."

This is so important. It makes her angry to not be at home, and that brings out the monster. So now we know the goal, the holy grail the monster searches for: home, not only a physical or emotional state, but a spiritual state.

"Tell me more about the life you would create within that spiritual state of home."

"It would be me and others, it would be like being one of a million molecules. I was the essence of what everything was."

Cheesecake has a little bit of "home" in it; this is where the bigness, the monster, is trying to get her to. Within the longing for cheesecake is the longing to reach a profound state, a taste of the transcendence that a near-death experience often gives. In both "cheesecake bliss" home and an overdose state, Francesca was detached from regular life. When she goes there, it gives her perspective on life. As she put it, "It is like being connected to something deeper while you are in the middle of life."

Concluding Thoughts

Housed within Francesca's criticism of her body is intense power. Like some women, her power is split off and becomes a critic and expresses itself by attacking the body. It uses criticism ("You are fat and ugly"), but the power behind it is another thing, a live ember, a great spirit. That power finds a place to live and tears her apart. It has always torn her apart, since she was a kid. Now it tears her apart about her weight.

This is an important point about critics. Sometimes they house great power, but the content is irrelevant. The power Francesca wields against herself is the deeper point. What she once fought with on the outside, she now uses to fight herself on the inside.

"If not for the drugs, I could have been something really big in my life, really big," Francesca says.

"You are meant for something big, and you are doing something really big by just living a normal life, because of everything you've had to survive. But I know you want more than that."

"I don't think most people would be able to survive what I've been through. It takes a very strong person to spend any significant time around me. I'm meant to be a great teacher. Why else would I have been through all these things?"

In Francesca's "ordinary" life, she has no place to be a warrior, a gladiator, a powerful shaman up against enormous forces. Where has she had those battles? In drugs, in prison, up against her own body. Her great, heroic battles are fought on the battlefield of the body. With a little grace and support, this pattern can change.

Chapter Thirteen

Faith: *Shak'n It Up*

～

"You can be in prison in many ways. It could be your
relationship, your job, anywhere. You have to break out."

F AITH IS SIXTY-TWO years old and is happy that after a lifetime of feeling dissatisfied with her weight, she's finally
been dropping pounds in the last few months.

"I'm just discovering how to have the discipline to exercise
and eat what I should."

Discipline is often regarded as a key to making successful
weight change. But there are reasons that focusing solely on
discipline can lead people astray. First, while the word *disci-*
pline has the same root as the word *disciple*, suggesting the relationship between a loving student and teacher, the actual *prac-*
tice of being disciplined is often accompanied by an attitude of
self-correction and chastisement, especially for those who were
raised in a more punitive culture or family environment. As a
result, many of us rightfully resist and even rebel against being
"disciplined" by not following through on our weight-loss strategy. Essentially, what looks like rebelling or derailing our efforts
may actually be a self-loving reaction to a punitive atmosphere
that really needs to change.

Second, as I have indicated, there are often deeper hungers

behind our hungers that motivate people to eat or grow in body size. When these motivations are not dealt with, people often blame themselves for not being sufficiently disciplined, as opposed to investigating these deeper motivations. In short, being more disciplined without regard for our true underlying hungers will rarely be sustainable.

"What kind of discipline have you found?" I ask.

"I have a big dog who needs to walk each day. He's a hundred and five pounds. I've always said I'm too busy to exercise after work. Now I'm making myself do that once in the morning and twice after work. I'm also trying to not eat much after five at night. I realize that I just don't need that much food. Whatever psychological reasons that caused me to gain so much weight have reversed themselves. I'm glad. People look at you when you are heavy and think, 'She has no control, no self-discipline.'"

Faith has a sense that she has conquered the problem, that after sixty-two years she has gotten over some problem and now she has integrated the discipline she needs.

"If I came to you and asked, 'Dear wise woman, please teach me what you have learned about discipline,' what would you say?" I am hoping to uncover Faith's deeper understanding, making more conscious the strengths and potential limits of her thinking.

"You have to understand what it *means* to have that discipline or what that discipline looks like. Because eating and not exercising is the opposite of discipline. For example, I would eat toast and butter at nine at night. I mean, I am from Wisconsin and I love butter. Or mashed potatoes, with lots of butter."

"Mmm, toast and butter, that's good," I say. We both laugh, acknowledging our common butter-love tribe.

"You're the Zen discipline master," I say. "'I just want some toast, I know there are things I need to do, but I just want some toast.' What would you say to me?"

"You have to know how to approach it, how to build that discipline into your life through structure. I have a very structured day, I have a dog, I go to work—"

"But what's happening during that time when you are sort of freewheeling? How can you turn that freewheeling time into structure? How can you structure it so you are not thinking so much about eating, food, and feeding whatever psychological need you are feeding?"

"Structure happens when you are more active than passive. It's passivity that is the problem," she says, as it occurs to her. Faith and I are already developing a deeper understanding of discipline—it's a fight against passivity.

"Ah," I say, "so it's structure and passivity."

"Yes, you have to monitor your own behavior."

I see her hand making a karate chop, indicating a communication that wants to be clear and direct.

"Give it to me straight, right between the eyes," I say, encouraging her, echoing the energy of her chop. "I'm pretty passive over here." I am taking on the role of the passive part of her, the part of her that she is in a conflict with, to further understand this inner conflict she is having.

She laughs. "I would grab you and shake you. I would be in your face."

"Wow, that's strong," I say, looking at her face as she moves toward me.

"But grabbing, shaking people doesn't work," she says. "You have to be open or willing to make the choice. You have to make choices, not be passive."

"I still want to get to know this part of you that would grab someone. Can you speak to me from that place?" I ask Faith to go back to the role-play where I represent the part of her that she wants to shake up. I am hoping to give Faith greater access to this antipassivity force that is now showing up in the impulse to grab and shake.

"Look, you're sixty-two years old," she says. "You've been overweight since you were fifteen or seventeen."

"I know, I just don't know what to do about it," I say, continuing to play my role.

"You have something you can do about it. You can make choices and you can change the way you live so that you don't just lay around eating. Between 6 and 9 PM, do something else."

I see the energy animating her as she delivers these thoughts, an energy that is a key to a deeper understanding of discipline, even something beyond discipline.

She says, "Do something about it. That's where I'm at. I can't afford to waste any more years of passivity. The first thing I need to do is take control over it. I have high blood pressure, high cholesterol, the whole range of stuff. I have been on antidepressants."

I say, trying to empathize, "It's time, you have been on antidepressants, you have high cholesterol. It's enough."

"It's time," she says.

"What else do you want to shake me up about? Wake me up, please continue. What else should I do with my life?" I again return to the role-play.

"Get out of the house."

"What do you mean, should I move?"

"Go out. Staying in the house, watching TV, encourages passivity," she says harshly, fiercely.

"How about the direction of my life? What else should I stop?" I ask these questions because many people, when they contact their deeper intelligence, have ideas beyond changing eating and exercise habits.

She laughs. "I have found that whenever I have traveled abroad, lived in different places, I immediately drop forty pounds. It just happens."

From Daily Discipline to Being Free

Something has changed; something has deepened. We just learned that traveling abroad is an effective weight-loss strategy, but it's quite different from what she had been calling discipline: trying not to eat late, going for a walk. This is a change that happens not by countering the everyday passivity she has spoken of so far; it is a change that happens automatically with a certain life change. These forty pounds get lost in a whole different paradigm.

"How does that work?"

"The environment changes. That's a great way to experience life, to understand life." She clears her throat, indicating deeper feelings.

"Ah, when you say 'it's time' to change your life, you mean really go far."

"It's about fear," she says. "You have to break through some fear barrier in order to get beyond the passivity."

"I feel it," I say, going back to the role. "What else should I break through, get beyond?"

"You should break out of prison," she says. "You can be in prison in many ways. It could be your relationship, your job, anywhere. You have to break out."

I can see that energy is now alive, at her disposal. We have released the genie of her deeper intelligence. It is no longer haunting her to not eat toast at night—it wants her to break free. While she is hungry to lose weight, she is even more hungry to be free in her relationships, her work—her life.

"I often find myself feeling imprisoned in my job. It is very intense and doesn't feel good."

"If you were to give me a message about this job, what would it be?"

"Join the Peace Corps," she says, clearly, congruently, as if she has had that answer waiting for a long time. She laughs. "Which is what I've been thinking for a while."

Even though Faith has been thinking regularly about changing jobs, it has never occurred to her that this may be a resolution to her unhappiness with her body. It has never occurred to her that even her desire to eat might be an expression of a hunger for a deeper change. Her earlier notion of discipline did not include this kind of resolution.

"Ah, don't just go outside, go outside of the whole box, the whole prison."

"Exactly, all those cultural forces that bombard people about who they are supposed to be, how they're supposed to live. When you are outside the culture, you don't have to buy into those. It is so much easier. I am planning, when I retire, to go into the Peace Corps. I know I would be happier in South Africa, even given the great struggles. These matter to me. I don't want to be here." Her eyes fill with tears. "That's when you find yourself, especially when you are alone. You are up against life, real life, and you have survived." She is brimming with passion, not the passion of criticizing herself, of trying to be more disciplined, but of feeling alive. "When you are abroad, you aren't expected to assimilate. It's not possible. There is so much freedom in that space between those two cultures. When I'm away, I see myself as a fringe dweller."

I can now see that the intelligence that fueled Faith's conviction about discipline was really about shaking her out of a kind of passivity—not the passivity of everyday life, but the passivity that prevents her from aligning with the kind of person she truly is, from living a life that is truly hers.

"You are a freedom fighter, fighting for your freedom."

"Anytime I make a big leap in my life, I don't allow myself to think of the what-ifs—I just move forward. If you start thinking about the fear, you're dead." She is laughing now, sitting up, interrupting, smiling, engaged. She is alive, animated.

"I love this aspect of you—it has the answer. There is an aliveness to it."

"Let me tell you, this has gotten me in a lot of trouble at work. It's got me hanging on by a thread."

Even when a life hunger is unconscious, it still lives. In this case, it still threatens to shake up Faith's job security.

"Yes, from one perspective your attitude threatens your security, but from another, that security builds prison walls. Shaking things up, breaking down prison walls, this may very well be the antidepressant your system needs."

Faith is a fringe dweller. She is capable of a life of service, of battling extraordinary challenges. But this great power in her has been co-opted, used to teach her discipline and fight her overeating. Deep down, this power is meant for so much more. It wants to shake up her life, break her free. And then, the weight just comes off. I decide to explore this with her a little bit more. She tells me about her history of travel and relocation.

"I left home the day after I graduated high school. I couldn't wait to get away, and I did, traveling to Africa. Then later, I moved to Africa. Then I went to Senegal, to the University of Jakarta. Up until last year, I was in a relationship for twenty-four years. We didn't always live together, but we were committed. After I left him, the discipline began. And I'm thinking about going into the Peace Corps. I'm good at implementing big projects."

"That shaker-upper—that's you."

"I am not identified with that, I don't see myself that way, I need to connect with that. Yes, that part doesn't have to think about dieting. She is a free person. I wonder how much the work of my life has taught me to conform to certain standards of behavior, versus this other side which wants to just get in the car and drive and sit in peace and just take it all in. I struggle with that."

"These are the two powers of your life: something that creates boxes and something that tries to break free." This is critical for any sustainable weight-loss effort Faith will make, because any program, plan, or discipline will likely also create a box. And where there is a box, when it comes to Faith, there is a freedom cry that is likely to be even stronger.

She continues, "When I was twelve years old, I remember we all piled in the car and went to Chicago. When I saw the suburbs and all those ticky-tacky suburbs and houses, I thought, 'I will never live that life. That's what everyone wants.'"

Faith didn't grow up in one of those ticky-tacky houses; she was raised by Catholic nuns. She might have preferred to be raised in a family, but the situation gave her the gift of being able to question that way of life. She might even sense that those houses can be too-small boxes.

"The breaking out," I say, "is even more powerful than the

discipline. The great power you use to break out can help you do so many other things." The diet, among other things, is a box that's too small for her.

A Toast-and-Butter Life

Faith tells me that her favorite food is butter. We begin an exploration of this hunger, the taste that she is looking for.

"What is it like to have toast and butter?"

"The texture—it's a visceral feeling."

"Here it is, some warm toast, butter melting and dripping into the little cracks." I am staying close to the visceral, the sense experience, in order to access her somatic intelligence.

"Oh yeah," she says, "it's soaking with butter."

"Here it is, take some. What is it like? What happens to you when you eat it?"

"It is a pleasure I feel. It is very satisfying."

"What kind of pleasure? Foot-rub pleasure? Lying-in-a-field pleasure?"

"Well, there also has to be salt—I don't eat unsalted butter. I mean, unsalted butter is good, but not the same. And it should be on something, like potatoes, soft and creamy. It's like baby food." Faith ignores my question about the kind of pleasure because she is still sensing the particulars of her experience. It's always a good sign when people stay close to their experience like this.

"And the little baby eats this warm, moist, creamy, slightly salty butter. What would the baby do?"

"It's like sucking my thumb. I did that until I was eleven years old." She found a way to self-soothe, and understandably, relied on it for a longer than usual amount of time. When she stopped, butter was a satisfying substitute. "I can just do this by myself. I don't need anything else, don't need to be there for anyone else, apologize for anything else."

Can you see the freedom? Guiltless pleasure. There isn't any discussion of whether this is right or wrong. It's prior to right and wrong. It's pre-box. This is her nirvana.

"I don't get lonely, I treasure that. But there is no security in butter, no income, no friends."

"But in the butter world, there are no questions about security, income, or friends."

"So, what is butter?" she asks.

"When you have butter, you experience a deep sense of your own nature, and no box. You need a butter life, a butter cure," I say. We both laugh. "The butter cure is that state of mind. The baby's state of mind—no thoughts, no fear, no need to be there for others, no guilt. No boxes. It's a state of absolute freedom."

"Empty mind," she says. "It's the essence of life." It's deeper than the freedoms of daily life, but a spiritual freedom.

"A reminder of the essence of life," I say. "Why should you break out? Because there are nuns that put you in boxes, as well as the memory of butter, which reminds you to break out and achieve what is possible as a human."

Concluding Thoughts

Faith is not just someone who sits back and feels peaceful; she has a huge hunger to break herself out of boxes. This is why she wants to go into the Peace Corps and take on big projects. She is a freedom fighter and a shaker-upper; her peace is not only being at ease, it is doing the breaking-out itself. When she's not free—working at a limiting job in the United States, for instance

—her power turns toward diet and exercise. She focuses on discipline and makes an enemy of her daily passivity. However, when she goes deeper and breaks out of her box and lives in another country, or changes a job, or ends a relationship, the weight comes off, and she uses her power for more far-reaching purposes.

Chapter Fourteen

Monica: *The Wounding Mother*

———

*"When I was little, and kids hurt me, I would want to go to my
mother, but she was one of the bigger bullies in my life."*

O NE OF THE saddest things about our society's value system
occurs when mothers damage their daughters by criticizing them about their weight. I'm not talking about a mother's
supportive suggestions, or creating mindfulness in one's family
about healthy choices and making healthy meals. I'm talking about
the ongoing, virulent criticism and shaming of a little girl's body
by the person they most need and trust.

Fortunately, a lot of awareness about the harm of this behavior has penetrated parents' consciousness over the last few decades. But there is still a generation of women whose mothers
believed that the best thing for their young daughters was to tell
them they had better diet or else they'd be fat, rejected, unhappy, and friendless.

As Monica says, "When I was little, and kids hurt me, I
would want to go to my mother, but she was one of the bigger
bullies in my life." Even though Monica is an adult, her mother
continues to inflict painful criticism on her when they talk.
Monica also suffers from anxiety attacks.

In our work together we explored what eating gives Monica

in terms of satisfying needs that are otherwise going unfulfilled, and ways for her to give herself what she needs in ways that are aligned with her conscious goals.

"When did you become aware of your weight?" I ask.

"I was five or six. I went to Catholic school, and my mother had to special-order the uniforms in my size, which was bigger than average. Then they were too long and had to be altered. My mom was really upset. She has had issues with weight her whole life, and that affected how she dealt with me.

"Because of my weight, my mom thought no one would like me, people would tease me, I wouldn't have any friends. I could tell that instead of empathizing with me, she was disgusted. My mom has always been caught up in how things make her look. I made her look bad, I didn't live up to her standards. I can't remember what she said, but I remember crying. My dad still has a picture of me sitting on his lap. My eyes were all swollen and puffy. From that age on, it escalated. She says she was trying to help me, but it hurt me."

A mother's disgust of her daughter's body enters the psyche with such fierce determination that it can impact the way a woman looks at her own body for a lifetime. Some women learn to "mother" themselves by trying to lose weight motivated by disgust and body shame for years to come. Instead of equating mothering to loving and nurturing and protecting, mothering becomes punishing, disgust-inducing, and shaming.

"As a kid, I became the class clown. I took on the role of entertainer. I had lots of friends and was popular, but it was also at the expense of myself, because I wasn't being true to myself. The entertainer wasn't really who I was. I would make a joke about my weight before anyone else could. Everyone thought I was a happy-go-lucky kid, but inside I was really unhappy and depressed. I always thought that if I ever let what was inside of me out, I was afraid I would never stop crying, that I would be miserable. That I might kill myself."

"I'm sorry you had to carry all that inside of you. When did your childhood sadness connect to thoughts of suicide?"

"I started thinking about it a lot in high school, when three different teenagers committed suicide in my community. I didn't really act on that until college. My family was Catholic, so I didn't want to hurt them by overtly killing myself. I thought if I got into an accident, then they would feel differently. I would drink and drive, and wake up in some other place and not know how I got there."

Monica's suicidality was in response to a psychic murder. A part of her was being killed off. A person's sense that they could kill themselves can actually be a positive sign that they have the capacity and determination to "end" an old life. With proper care and empowerment and consciousness, that capacity can help them turn their whole life around and not harm themselves. Monica was eventually able to do that.

"It's a kind of suicide," I say, "to deny oneself, to put oneself away and be the clown."

"Yes, and I got tired of playing the game. I felt like I was wearing this mask. It is bad enough being in pain, but then there was an agony of not even being myself. I acted for so long that I didn't even know who I was. The one thing I did know about myself was that I was overweight."

Knowing only this one thing about herself is a terrible fixation for Monica because her weight, remember, is being "mothered" by disgust and shame, crippling the development of other areas of her life and soul.

"I recently lost some weight and asked my mother, "Do you

think it really helped me, have I lost the weight?" I still had more to lose, but I wanted her approval. She only said, 'I'm concerned about your health. Obviously, losing that ninety pounds has backfired on you.'"

"This is so important," I say. "Your mother's words are about trying to help, but the tone and attitude betray another message. It is hurtful and shaming, and so hard to protect yourself because of the double message."

When a person as influential as a mother consistently communicates with double messages—*I care about you, but am disgusted by you*—it is essential that the person begin to see these double messages. Otherwise they buy into the first message, *I care about you*, and become blind to the second, *I'm disgusted by you*, even though the second message still wounds. If this doesn't get clarified, the person can live a life where they get hurt, over and over, but are not free to trust their own perceptions and experience of being mistreated, hurt, or abused. This lack of self-trust is part of the core of shame.

"About two years ago," Monica says, "I was supposed to have sinus surgery. I didn't do it, but I did lose about ninety pounds in preparation for the surgery. The doctor was really impressed, and supportive of my weight loss.

"And then recently, because I've been sick with a sinus infection, I told my mother that I needed to see the doctor. She asked, knowing that I had gained back weight, 'Has he seen you *lately?*' in this tone like, 'Oh my God, the way you look now.' I canceled my appointment and went to a different doctor, even though I would rather have gone to him."

"I would feel ashamed if someone said that to me," I say. "A lot of women avoid going to the doctor because of the way doctors talk to them about their weight."

It's true, many women don't go to doctors because they don't want to get on the scale and have the doctor make a cold or critical comment. It's simply too painful.

"Definitely. I get afraid to go to doctors. Even when I go to my ear, nose, and throat doctor, he makes comments about my weight. When I did lose the ninety pounds, I felt so much better. But I still had more weight to lose. And I thought, 'To come this far and still have this much to go.' I just gave up."

Recovery of the Self

To help Monica recover or establish trust in her own experience, she must connect with her deeper feelings and reactions to the insults, criticisms, shame, and disgust. We return to some of her painful experiences and hold a space for the truth of her feelings to arise and be witnessed. This is the way shame gets healed.

"Let's go back to what happens when your mom made a statement like, 'Has the doctor seen you like this?' What happens to you?"

"I thought, 'Oh my God, I can't go back to him. He will be disappointed, and I'm disappointed in myself.' And then I go back to all the hurtful things my mother used to say, and I just want to wring her neck."

Monica makes a gripping, choking hand motion, an instance of her body communicating with me. I engage with this physical expression, knowing that the truth of her reaction to her mother is arising somatically.

"Let's go into that hand motion. Make that motion again and feel that reaction you have."

She makes the choking motion again, saying, "I just want her to stop. We've done this for thirty-three years. I'm thirty-nine now. It's been an issue almost my whole entire life. And now that I'm a mother, it is even more hurtful. When you're a mother, there is so much unconditional love. I feel it, why didn't my mother? When I was little, and kids hurt me, I would want to go to my mother, but she was one of the bigger bullies in my life."

"Where else do you feel that gripping feeling?" I ask in order to build a deeper and more sustaining relationship with the intelligence of her body.

"I feel it in my throat and in my mouth. I am clenching my jaw. In my throat, it's like a big lump, and when I swallow, I can really feel it. It is like a sore throat when I try to speak, it's almost painful."

I am not surprised that it is in the throat, because she wants to wring someone's throat, but she also wrings her own throat, cuts off her own authentic self-expression. (It's not uncommon for aggression to be internalized, taken out on one's self, when it is not free to express itself outwardly.) I give her a small pillow so she can externalize her ferocity. She grabs it and starts to cry.

"Stop! Just stop! It doesn't bother me anymore. I say that, but it does."

She thinks she shouldn't be bothered. She wants to get beyond this reaction. So many people say, "Get over it," but it keeps happening, and inside of her is the thing that might be able to end it, this voice that says "Stop, just stop!"

Shame almost always discourages us from feeling the full expression of our pain, anger, or resistance. People are told that these feelings are indicators of a lack of psychological health when actually it's quite the opposite: freedom from shame's suppression.

I ask, "Can you close your eyes for a moment? When you hear that voice that says 'stop,' how loud is it?" I am hoping Monica will now broaden her experience of her truth, moving from the body to sound and voice. I am hoping she feels herself in her body, in her movement, in her voice, in her ears—everywhere.

"It's like a scream."

"Let's try it together, that loud."

Monica has a big voice and I want to support her reaction, her expression.

"Stop already!" she says with a little bit more volume. "But, I don't know that I can yell like that. And besides, she doesn't really hear me. Like when I tell her things that happened when I was a kid, she says, 'I never said that. That isn't true.' So in addition to the initial hurt, she makes me crazy by denying it."

"What would crazy look like? Would you be screaming or comatose?" I ask because the word *crazy* often indicates a freedom of feeling or expression beyond a person's comfort zone. People often feel crazy when a situation is crazy making, meaning when they are given mixed messages, when they are put in double binds. (For example, "I will make you angry, but you must get not angry.")

"I don't have a whole lot of tears left, I don't really know. Maybe yelling, or lying on the floor in a ball. Maybe wanting to scream, but having a hard time getting the words out. And then just rolling around on the floor going crazy."

"Like this," I say, and I contort my face and I groan and scream. "Stop! Don't you hear, don't you listen?"

We go back to using the role-playing method. I pretend to be her mother, hoping that Monica can find the power of her voice now that we've explored it further.

I say, "What? I am just caring for you, what should I stop?"

"But you aren't caring, you hurt me."

"I am just here trying to help."

"I can't do this anymore," she says while shaking my hand. "You lie, you make my life worse, and I can't do it anymore. You are my mom and you hurt me more than anyone ever hurt me." She is shaking me harder. "Stop," she says even louder, "it has to stop." Her face is red, I see her eyes grow big. I see this huge voice and power that's beginning to come out.

To help her further, I switch. I speak her words. I say, "Stop, stop, stop. I want to wring your neck. Why aren't you going away? No matter what I do, you are still there. You are driving me crazy."

"That's it," she says. "I feel like I'm going in circles, over and over."

"I am going crazy, get me out of here, I can't stand it!" I start saying, with panic and mania. I get wild.

"People don't know that is inside of me," Monica says, beginning to get closer to her true self.

"Do you know that it is inside of you?" I ask. I think of the clown role she played as a child, to be accepted, to deal with all the judgments her mother put on her, and how that obscured her own self-discovery.

"I don't think I know what is inside of me. I think it is a strength, but I am afraid of it. It is a spirit."

"What are you afraid of?"

"If I really said what I had to say, it would change my whole life. Everything would be different, not just my relationship with my mom, but everything. I would pack my bags, leave my husband. It would be an everything kind of change. And now, because I am a mom, I have to contain it."

When people come in contact with a long-suppressed true self, there is a sense that everything will have to change. In a way, that's true, because the change they are about to make will reorient their relationship to themselves, other people, and the world around them.

"If you would let it out, everything would change. Feel the energy of it again."

She makes a fist and tenses her jaw.

"Dear spirit," I say to her, "you would wipe everything clean, change absolutely everything."

"I would start over and be the person I was meant to be. I don't know if I know what that is."

"Dear spirit, you must know the kind of person Monica really is. Please tell me who she is."

"I think it's there. It's lost but I think it can be found. But there's a fear in finding it. I am pretty adaptable, I can take things. I can go the rest of my life being this way."

Monica is close to standing in her power and a deep self-knowledge about who she is, yet fear and adaptability are still working against her. She switches back and forth between an old identity and a new one, a truer one. Perhaps a dialogue between the part of her who wants to come out, who wants to not get lost, with the one who is frightened will help her awareness and clarity grow. We proceed.

I say, "You have contained me, but I can't be contained. I have never been totally contained. I have always been here."

"I am afraid of you," she says. "I need to keep you inside, I don't know what you would do to others in my life."

"You are right to be afraid of me. I would sacrifice it all, I would change it all."

"I don't know if I can take you on right now."

I switch roles again, seeing if Monica can get in touch with the part of her that has been contained.

I say, "I need to box you up, contain you."

"You're hurting my spirit, my body," she answers.

"I don't know what to do, I'm too afraid to let you out."

"Some of it needs to be let out," she says, "I can't take how I feel anymore."

"How will you do that? I am afraid. You are giving me panic attacks, making me feel so bad. How can we do that?"

"Even though I am so strong, I am afraid to do that," she says.

I feel an intimacy developing between Monica and me, and Monica and herself. We know who she is and where she is in her story, her personal development. She is negotiating with two parts of herself. Wrestling with this inner conflict is critical to the next steps in her development.

I say, "Dear spirit, can we let out a little bit now and still make it safe for me?"

Monica responds, "I think I could let a little bit of it out and enclose the other part of me, wrap myself in myself."

I give her a pillow and ask her to wrap herself around it.

"I am holding on really tight but it's not to stifle it. I am holding you, please don't go away. I know I am holding you tightly. I will let you become freer soon. I know I have to, I just need to hold you first and get to know you."

I feel the intimacy she is developing with the power inside her. It's absolutely gorgeous. This is a great dialogue between a part of her that contains her, and something totally free and unknown.

I say, "The spirit itself has its own life. When someone puts it down, it gets crazy and angry. For some part of you, it's worth dying if it, the spirit, can't get free." I am remembering the suicidality that arose earlier in her life and our interaction. What was once the dangerous suicidality that arose earlier in

Monica's life is now a power she can use to make an ending and a new beginning.

"That spirit has always been here," she says, "even before I was here, before I was alive. I think it will be there even after I die, so that's a comfort. Part of the spirit got locked inside of me, half is free."

"Could you consciously let that spirit out, to make the relationship with yourself a little bit easier?" I ask.

"This spirit in me is not a fat, ugly girl like I've been told. I know it is not what my body is. If I could slowly release it, I might really be successful at dieting."

"Dear spirit," I say, wanting to access this new intelligence, "I'm sitting here thinking, why am I getting heavy again? Please help me. What do you think?"

"My spirit doesn't really care, it just accepts me as I am. It's not what it's about, it is accepting. It already knows the beauty in me."

"If you want to lose weight, the doorway is to not care," I say. "That is the spirit's way, an acceptance way. It is not an agenda, it is a giving over, a giving up, so that the spirit can express itself. That is the doorway. You may have to go with the spirit. I don't know if you should lose weight or gain weight, but how you approach yourself is key. You must see the beauty in you, the beauty you are, like the spirit sees it."

This is such a profound insight for so many women who are dying to get smaller. It's truly a paradox. Trying to lose weight is often an act of nonacceptance, exactly the opposite of the power that is needed. "Not caring" was the release of her spirit that ended up playing a key role in Monica's growth in the years that followed our work together.

Monica's Update

Years later, Monica wrote to me. "After working with you, I realized that shame and guilt was not mine to carry." Society's and her mother's messages had sold her on believing she should feel ashamed. "But because I had been carrying extra weight in the form of shame and guilt, I was also carrying physical weight. *That* was mine to carry. I had to sit with it, and accept my role in gaining the weight. It was also my responsibility to understand how all the guilt, shame, abuse, and pain shaped who I had become physically and emotionally.

"I was in an abusive relationship during this time, because I had settled. I thought he was what I deserved. But as I began to embrace the darkness and sadness within me, to feel and grieve, I began to shed the emotional weight, and that began with leaving and eventually divorcing my husband. The weight lost from that relationship was such a relief. I felt I could breathe again. I felt light and empowered."

Divorce is seldom easy or painless, and before Monica felt light and empowered, she describes hitting bottom and sitting with her pain, something she "had to endure to find my strength. I didn't try to climb my way out. I had to sit in the darkness and embrace it and to give myself grace." She had to accept herself as she was, shadow and all.

"As I shed the emotional weight, I was proud of the person I was becoming. I accepted myself completely. Not only the emotional, but physical. Because of our work together, David, I accepted my own body, a body I had been told by others was not beautiful, was not healthy, was not accepted. About six months after coming to this acceptance, I began to shed the physical weight of my body, and I was doing so without any restrictive dieting or exercise. I was happy, and food no longer became a focus or a protective factor. Over the course of that year I lost a little over a hundred pounds. I liked the way I was feeling physically. I began to live a healthier lifestyle for me, and not to appease others.

"I got to the point where I decided to seek a goal weight, a number for myself. That's when the weight loss slowed and over the last year I have been losing and gaining the same twenty pounds, which I find interesting. I am exploring the reasons behind this pattern."

I shared with Monica that it might be related to the strength and power Monica finds in "not caring," in accepting herself as she is. Her body may be registering that goal weight, that number, as a kind of caring that is too aligned with trying to please others. It may also evoke the old patterns of resistance around dieting.

The arbitrariness of numbers, and their ability to muddy the waters of happiness and self-acceptance, is something she's continuing to learn and relearn, especially after having what many people consider to be a significant birthday. "As I turned fifty, I realized I am no longer a number on a scale or my age. I am so much more than a number." Monica's growth has also shown up in her emotional life. She is now in a healthy relationship for the first time. "He is successful, intelligent, and loving, and he came along when I finally realized I am deserving of that."

Chapter Fifteen

Kelly: *Getting By with* More *(Instead of Less)*

"I've never had exactly what I want. I tell my kids, 'Don't let anyone get in your head and tell you to be different from who you really are.'"

MANY OF US are taught, from an early age, that we are not the author of our own lives. Our own impulses, desires, and needs are subject to others' determination of whether they are worthy, valid, or appropriate. And sometimes, even if they are deemed worthy, the authorities that be are unwilling to be challenged or resisted. They are in control; they must be "honored."

When Kelly was a child, her parents taught her, "Don't speak unless spoken to." She was also taught that it was disrespectful to talk back or disagree, and that she should be happy to have whatever was given to her, even if it was insufficient, or worse, caused her harm.

Too often, as was the case for Kelly, we are taught to sacrifice our desires to the egos and power trips of parents and other authority figures. A teacher of mine once told me that a child who is made to share before they can declare "This is mine" may be unable to give without resentment for years to come, if they can bring themselves to give at all. Learning to go for what we want, to grab hold of our deepest desires, to dream big, and to believe in our yearnings and longings can take a back seat to the allegedly nobler pursuits of giving to others, being unselfish, or serving someone else's purpose.

Kelly describes herself as perfectionistic. "I never liked to read aloud in school. I feared getting called on. I felt such pressure that I couldn't even focus. I could read on my own. Despite that, I always did well in school." However, she did not continue her education after high school, even though she deeply wanted it, but she felt pressure to accommodate herself to the authority of higher education's schedules and approaches, and that didn't work for her.

Kelly grew up in a home that was both wonderful and joyful, and agonizing and abusive. When she didn't behave according to her parents' expectations, they retaliated with violence. Her mother slapped her, and if her father was crossed, he would do much more.

"My mom—she didn't hesitate. It didn't matter where you were. If I was sassy, at home, with friends, or in a store, she would slap me across the face. My dad was the strong disciplinarian. He wouldn't deal with things when they came up, he would wait. He was pretty physical with my brother and older sister, not really so much with me. I saw what he did to my brother and sister. I once saw him kick my brother right in the stomach."

When her mother drank too much, which was often, she turned belligerent and rowdy. Her father responded by beating her. Kelly used to stand between her parents and entreat her father: "She doesn't know what she's doing, she doesn't know what she's saying. You're hurting her. You're going to get in trouble for this."

And yet Kelly still has some good childhood memories: fishing trips and barbecues. As far back as she can remember, her parents' rules denied her own power and authority. Did she ever feel like she had any? Did she have an opportunity to even notice the loss? Perhaps not consciously, but her behavior around food shows a strong drive to go after exactly what she wants (finally!)—to ask for it, to disagree with anyone or anything who tells her she's wrong, and to voice her disappointment with anything that falls short, instead of defaulting to a weak approximation of gratitude. Ideally, Kelly would be able to use this existing personal authority and sense of entitlement in all areas of her life, not just around eating. Unless this is resolved, it will cause her ongoing suffering, both in the ways she does not follow the dictates of her own authority, and in the ways the internalized authority of others gets used against her in areas that undermine her stated goals, sabotaging any diet program she takes on.

This is one reason why traditional diet programs don't work: their very design separates people from their autonomy, authority, and power. Many weight-loss experts insist that people just need to be more "responsible" and "accountable" and "disciplined." They don't see or acknowledge the complexity of what's going on at a psychological level: that many women are not just fighting their habits or hungers, they're resisting the old authority figures who told them to be silent, to not talk back, to make do, and to be grateful for and satisfied by whatever paltry allotment came their way.

"Then I got married. I didn't realize how controlling my father was until I married my husband. I pretty much married my father. He's controlling and physically violent." Like many parents who vow that their children will have a better childhood than their own, Kelly found some solace in deciding that her children would not suffer her fate. She wanted them to embody the authority that she was denied.

"I raised my kids to think that they can talk back and speak up for themselves. If my child came home complaining about a teacher, I would take them to talk to that teacher. I wanted them to know that they could confront authority figures as long as they did so with respect."

Kelly also notes that her coworkers see her as having "so much more authority than I really have." There's a disconnect that echoes the way her parents disconnected her from her power. She identifies with not having the authority.

Weight Wrestling

Kelly has struggled with her weight since she was twelve years old.

"It was the summer before sixth grade. My body was changing. I could usually wear clothes from one school year into the next, but not this time. I'd always been a thin kid, but now I had a belly. That was the year that I got my first bra. My dad came home from work with a friend, and they were sitting at the kitchen table. My mom took my bra out of the bag, and said, 'Look at what we did today.'"

"It would have been hard to say, 'Mom, back off.'"

"That would not have been tolerated."

Because Kelly's mother strictly enforced her children's silence with slaps and more, Kelly didn't say anything while her privacy was violated, humiliating her in front of her father and his friend. She also knew she couldn't risk her even more volatile father's anger.

To be humiliated in front of others and have no one on your side—seeing, caring, and defending—is like being stripped naked in public. How can one stand in their own authority when they cannot say what is right and wrong for them, when they can't say

"Ouch, that hurts" or "No, that is not okay with me." If this core experience of a person's integrity is not protected, they may never be able to freely consent when any pressure is put upon them until they can reclaim their authority at this fundamental level. Kelly's struggles with her weight didn't become extreme until her two children were born. As an adult, Kelly has learned that "I can lose weight by eating salads and drinking water, but it's just a temporary thing." She was involved in an exercise program until recently, when she injured her ankle.

"My husband doesn't understand it. I don't eat a lot of junk food or drink sodas all day. But I've noticed that no matter what comes up for me, food is always the answer. If I am having a really bad day, I'll have a taco with sour cream on it. If it's been a really good week and we're going out to dinner, I'll have a baked potato with everything on it. When my son got his driver's license, I thought, 'I want to fix him a really nice dinner.'"

Food is the answer, but to what question?

"Every meal is a battle," Kelly says. "My hunger is a state of war." She considers herself lazy for not packing and bringing a healthy lunch to work. But if she did that, she wouldn't get to engage the inner battle in the cafeteria arena. "I can go to the cafeteria for a salad, but their salads are disgusting. I might have made really good decisions about breakfast, but then by lunch someone around me has some French fries, and I think, 'Boy, those smell good. That's what I need to get through this afternoon.' I'll go down to the cafeteria and look at the fries, go back and forth inside my head." I see this as Kelly in the constant conflict of trying to connect with the authority she lost as a young child.

She calls herself lazy and attacks herself for making

unhealthy decisions at the same time that she claims her authority by doing what she wants, eating something counter to her weight-loss goals.

Kelly's battle with food was a mirror for the battle she was unable to fully engage with outer authorities. She reached for food as an assertion, as if to say, "This is what I want. You can't tell me what to do. I don't care what you think." Some people, like Kelly, need to win the diet battle in a way that seems counterintuitive: winning means defeating the diet program and declaring their authority and autonomy.

Come Out, Come Out, Wherever You Are: Outing the Inner Authority

Who is this authority on the other side of her eating and dieting battle? Who makes her diet? Whose program is it, anyway? Why should she go along with it? Why not stand in the way like she did for her mother? Why not treat herself like she treats her kids, and support herself in standing up to this stupid authority? Instead, she is embroiled in a battle that causes her daily humiliation, conflict, confusion, and self-criticism.

You can see the bind. She fights this battle to engage with her own authority, to connect to it. But right now, to win means to eat things that are seemingly unhealthy. How can she proceed? Is it a win-lose, or is there a possible win-win? Yes, there is —but first she must integrate her authority into the part of herself that is not the critic. That is the first step, one she needs to take to make decisions that are deeply and truly life-affirming.

"Some people will go home and say, 'I need a margarita.' I don't do that, but I will say, 'I need a vanilla latte.' To have the latte or not is one decision, but then I go back and forth: decaf or not, skim milk or not, sugar or not. I'd never choose an artificial sweetener, because the chemicals are worse for you." She laughs. "I settle on the skim milk. Then I think, 'I like the other one better. Let's have that fight for a minute or two.'" It seems exhausting.

I suggest that we role-play. I want to further observe the way her urge to reclaim her power manifests around food. I want to make her battle with her diet program more conscious. I begin by echoing the voice of her hunger.

"Here we are," I begin, "we're going to the cafeteria. Those French fries sure look good. *Mmm*, I sure could use some French fries."

"You shouldn't have those French fries," Kelly replies. "They're bad for you, they're going to make you store fat. And potatoes are bad for you—you don't need the carbs. Plus, if you have the French fries, you are going to have dip."

"Mmm, I do want dip for them, now that you mention it," I say.

She laughs and laughs. I switch to the other side of the battle, the diet-conscious role.

"Then have a salad, you can have dip on the salad," I say.

"I don't want to have salad," Kelly says, "I want the French fries, they smell good." She goes on. "Then I'll compromise and have chicken strips. It's kind of like chicken breast, and it's not deep fried." Kelly is practicing not giving in by negotiating for what she wants. I am hoping she learns to do this in other areas of her life.

"I don't want you to have chicken strips, I want you to have salad," I say.

"Then I'll have the salad with the chicken strips diced up on it," Kelly rebuts.

"I don't want you to have chicken strips. They have the carbs and extra fat."

"I really want that deep-fried flavor."

"You'll have to get over that," I say, "I'm not open to you having deep-fried flavors. Salads are what you'll have to eat."

"Okay, then they really have to be good. Is there boiled egg on it, blue cheese, maybe crumbled bacon?"

We both laugh as the inner battle becomes more conscious and as Kelly gets more creative and freer in standing for what she wants. A joy arises when a person's truer but more forbidden voice emerges.

"I walk around the cafeteria and say, 'I don't want that, I shouldn't have that. If I really need a hamburger, I won't order the cheese, or the bun, or the lettuce or the tomato, and I'll eat it that way. I won't get the fries, and it satisfies something." It's a far cry, I will soon learn, from the deluxe, loaded burgers of her childhood that she truly desires.

When it comes to nourishment, Kelly is engaged in constant negotiations. Her impulse to be satisfied arises, and she acknowledges it, and at the same time, it provokes an internalized authority that works against her. Reenacting this battle, the battle of her childhood and life, is exactly what we all do—find a place to manifest the struggles that we haven't worked out, maybe with food, maybe in relationship with another, or maybe with some form of addictive tendency. Seeing this strange but very human 'perfection' helps keeps shame away. And, in keeping shame away, it becomes easier to resolve.

These internalized authorities often show up as inner criticism. They are a major source of low self-esteem, of not liking or loving oneself. Many women have internalized this criticism about their bodies and eating habits, conforming to the objectification they experience in the outer world. If this problem is not addressed first, any diet program ends up in the wrong hands and will rarely be successful.

Going further, Kelly needs to confront this inner critic, this authority thief. She needs to steal its authority, make it her own. We continue role-playing.

I continue, "Dear critic, who thinks you know better than me, why do you think I reach for French fries, chicken strips?"

"The word *lazy* keeps rolling through my mind. If the lazy part of me didn't get in the way, the smart part of me would make salads and bring them with me."

"Is that your whole opinion of me? Even when I bring a salad, I want to go to the cafeteria and look at yummy things that I want. Why do you think I am still interested in those foods?"

"Maybe because other people can have them. Other people can sit around and eat Doritos and sugar-laden pop all day, and they're either real thin, or they just don't care."

"You are really critical of me. I think you just don't like me."

"You are lazy. You don't take the time to shop, take the time to fix the dinner and fix the salad. The house is not as clean as it should be. The lazy part of me when I come home just wants to sit down. I should mow the lawn and trim the flowers and finish the painting. I should get my oil changed. Do my homework sooner than I do. Update my résumé."

"You are not a very smart critic," I say. "The only reason you can think of is that I am lazy. You have watched me all these years, and you can't think of anything else. You don't see my interests, my need for happiness and rest. You are sharp, challenging, but not very bright. You have a one-track mind, you stick to it. Your critique has never helped, has never led to any sustainable change, but you stick to it."

My fierce stance moves Kelly to take her own side; she goes back to supporting the part of her that wants to eat what she wants, the part that resists her critical internalized authority.

"I am not going to have salad, leave me alone. No wonder I can't sleep. You keep me up all night with all the things I haven't done."

"Well, you need to do those things."

"Well then, you're fired," Kelly says.

"You are going to fire me?"

"If I thought that I had that authority, yes, I would get rid of you."

Kelly is contemplating stepping into her authority, of taking charge of her life, of usurping the old guard.

Life brings out the best in us—or shall I say, it brings out *us*. Nature has her beauty and perfect symmetry from birds and worms and seeds and rains to each moment of our life. This symmetry guides us toward ourselves and our role.

We have to trust that once she integrates her authority into an inner loving witness, she will do what is good for her, best for her, healthy for her.

Make Me One with Everything

So what is Kelly truly hungry for? If she were aligned with her own authority, what would she reach for? As I spoke about in the introduction, our hunger for life can be discovered in our hunger for the foods we desire; we simply need to learn to ask.

I ask Kelly to focus more directly on eating, to engage with what she desires, without the mediation of the inner critic telling her what she should want.

"What would be the most forbidden food? What would be the most satisfying?"

"Probably a cheeseburger. It would have everything on it. When I was growing up, we would have these big homemade hamburgers with big buns. We made the hamburger patties with garlic powder, seasoned salt, chopped tomatoes, diced onion, egg —almost like a meat loaf, plus everything on it."

"When you say everything, what do you mean?"

"Cheddar cheese. Tomatoes, mayonnaise, mustard, ketchup, on top of a nice beef patty, nothing too thin, drippy, kind of running down your arm. Pickles, not relish, it's got to be a dill pickle, not those sweet sliced pickles. My dad was a sandwich eater. He never just had a bologna sandwich, it would have everything on it."

"What's so good about having everything on it? Imagine that you prepare that hamburger just the way you want it. And then what if I said, 'Can't we leave the mayonnaise off?'"

"The mayonnaise mixes with the ketchup and the mustard and they make a flavor. It's not the mayo or ketchup or mustard itself, it's how they combine to get a flavor you can't get any other way."

"Can't you leave off the bun?"

"You have to have a bun. It doesn't taste like a hamburger without the fresh bread. It's the package."

"Why pickles? Can't you let go of the pickles?"

"I could live without the pickles, but they are part of the flavor. They would be missing. It all has to be there!" We are thoroughly enjoying Kelly's ease and passion in arguing against compromising what she truly wants.

"Now imagine if we prepared it. Here it is, runny, it's got the mayonnaise. Tell me about it in a way that makes me want it."

"It really is beautiful, how you can get all this on a round piece of bread with all those colors. And when you bite into it, you get all these flavors, not just one. It was the best of my childhood: the fishing trips and barbecues."

"What is it like to know exactly what you want in every detail?"

"If you feed a craving and it's not exactly what you want, then it won't work, it's not going to fulfill it. You'll eat more because you're not satisfied. If you have the opportunity to have all of those extra things, then you should experience all those things. You should have that hamburger exactly the way you want it." She emphasizes her point by making a karate-chop motion.

"Tell me more about having exactly what you want, not leaving anything out."

"I've never had exactly what I want. I tell my kids, 'Don't let anyone get in your head and tell you to be different from who you really are.' And yet, I know how prone to compromising I am. I've believed that it's more important that others are happy, even with my kids, who are now adults."

"I've never had exactly what I want"— these words shake me with their power, clarity, and insight.

A good compromise can only occur when both parties are clear on exactly what they want at the outset. Anything else is a sacrifice, the sacrifice her parents demanded.

"Know and state exactly what you want," I say. "You may not end up with it, but you have to state it and know it."

I encourage Kelly to take this exploration on as a kind of yoga practice, asking, "Is this exactly what I want? What's missing?" She can ask this about her interactions with her husband, with her kids, at her job. "Ask this of everything in your life.

You'll find that almost everywhere in your life, there is a thief that says, 'You can get by with this, a little less.'"

Many things get silenced in childhood, but for Kelly, it was "This is exactly what I want."

I suggest that her first step is to eat whatever she wants. Not forever, get whatever you want for at least a few weeks, when you want it. The discipline is that you must not stop yourself. If you want cheese, you must get the cheese. If you think you want French fries, you must get the French fries. You can't say that you can only have some.

Kelly's Growth

Kelly later told me that the more freedom she gave herself to get the hamburger she wanted, the less hungry she became for them. She decided to get by with more, not less, and she began to eat less, not more. This is not an uncommon paradox around dieting.

And she took on two tasks to 'get what she wanted.' The first involved repainting a wall a color she wanted. Previously she had given in to her husband and family about the color. Some of her family wanted an off-white color that was more blue-green; she wanted an off-white color that was more red. You might think this distinction is rather small; in fact, that's why I find it so significant. But for Kelly standing for what she really wanted, even in this seemingly small way, was breaking free from an old authority, one that silenced her.

The second involved planning to go back to school—something she let go of to prioritize being a wife and mother. She didn't continue her education after high school, even though she deeply wanted it, because she felt pressure to accommodate herself to the authority of higher education's schedules and approaches, and that didn't work for her. Now she could stand for her own way, her own approach. She knew what she wanted and how she wanted to do it. She no longer needed to be deprived of getting a college education because giving up her authority was too big a cost. Her authority wasn't for sale.

I could feel the power, pride, and life flowing through her as she announced this decision to me.

Who would have thought going back to school could be a diet program? Who would have thought repainting a wall could be part of a diet program? Kelly educated me, taught me exactly how it could be true.

Chapter Sixteen

Sinead: *Authenticity Rules*

*"I am extremely strong. I am stubborn beyond words. I am
the master of doors. I control the openings, and I control that
freedom, and my strength must not be misjudged."*

WOMEN ARE SOCIALIZED from childhood to be accommodating, to make things easy for the people around
them, whether it's by smiling and nodding while listening to
people talk, or by acting calm and pleasant while a man is making unwelcome sexual advances. Most of the time, the behavior
is automatic. It's not driven by conscious thoughts like, "If you
don't act this way, you may be punished." Messages range from
reproving remarks, to subtle shunning, to hostile attack. These
terms often keep women penned in by institutionalized sexism.
But even if the outward, often unconscious behavior goes with
the flow, the body knows exactly what's going on and rebels.
How is a rebellion understood when its signals are not decoded?

Sinead's story is a profound example of these dynamics.
When this Irish woman was eleven years old, a trusted and charismatic clergy member molested and raped her over a period of
months. When she eventually told her parents and the community about his criminal behavior—ceasing to be accommodating—a heroic act within the vastly unequal power dynamics
of child-adult, female-male, and layperson-clergy—she was

vilified and shamed at every level, from her father, to the congregation, her schoolteachers, the police, the media, her schoolmates, and even her therapist, who put her on sedating drugs and suggested she was a seductress. The bishop himself, when he found out, told Sinead that she was ruining the priest's life by reporting him.

Like so many women, one of the ways her body responded to this excruciating persecution was a pattern of starving herself and then gaining excess weight. Sinead continues, so many years later, to be persistently haunted by her weight; she views her large body as an intense object of self-hatred and shame. She has also not left her house in seventeen years. Whenever she has tried to venture out into the world, she experiences vertigo, a symptom that also crops up when she's home.

When Sinead and I first speak, she tells me that she had previously worked with a therapist over a couple of years.

"What did you work on with your therapist?"

"He tried to help me get out of the house. The goal was to get me to walk a short distance down my driveway. It was never really successful."

"What's so good about staying at home?"

"No one ever asked me that."

This is one deadly impact of shame. Rather than her former therapist believing in Sinead's natural intelligence—an intelligence that resisted the therapist's counsel—they looked at Sinead as pathological, as someone needing fixing or correction to overcome her resistance, to overcome her natural intelligence. However inadvertently and well intentioned these efforts are, they still teach a person to not trust themselves. That's the cost shame demands we pay.

"If I try to push, if I try to do things, I feel dizzy. I can't lean my head back without placing it on a soft pillow. When I walk, I feel like a drunk person. The fascinating or frightening part is that this thing is so unpredictable, and it has a life of its own."

"That's a great phrase," I say, connecting the symptom to Sinead herself, providing distance for reflection by talking to her about herself using the third person. "'It has a life of its own.' *Sinead's body* has a life of her own. The symptom doesn't have a lot of flexibility in it: you can't go left too much this way, too much that way. In other words, parts of Sinead have very little flexibility in her—in the best sense, meaning she can't be pulled off course and follow sexism's accommodating dictates."

"Yes. Recently I felt I have much to do around the house. But then I became overcome with tiredness. My dizziness became so intense. I thought, 'I didn't choose this, this is not what I want to do.'"

"That's where your process is doing its dance, something you talked about earlier, about being very accommodating: 'I used to accommodate, or give myself away, or bend, or put on a face for other people.' You'd try to be more available to other people, although you were feeling like, 'No, damn it, I can't be something for somebody else anymore. I can't do that.' You may not have said the words or changed your actions, but your symptoms pushed back. Your body is saying that your journey has one direction. You have to be true to yourself, you have to follow it home. You can't afford to stop on the way. The demand of the soul is so strong, often expressed through the body, and yet we're human. We can't line up with our souls a hundred percent. We do bend. We go this way, we go that way, we have other needs we have to wrestle with. Nonetheless, the soul can be inflexible. It's like, 'Nope, true north, period. Home is the only way.' It will insist on that."

This is partly why the plan to get Sinead to walk down her driveway wasn't going to work. Sinead was on a journey toward a powerful authenticity. Pleasing anyone—a therapist, her family, or the culture at large—or doing things to appear more socially acceptable was a fight against the best of her, a strategy doomed to fail.

"When I think about going somewhere," Sinead says, "I think about other people seeing me. If I really wanted to meet a friend out in the world, would my body stop me from doing that? The feeling of shame and shyness and the feeling of having failed, would it stop me? Definitely, definitely, yes."

"So if you desired that connection, would it hold you back?"

"Yes."

"That's a clear yes, without hesitation. There's strength in that. All of you is lined up behind that yes. You wouldn't move, even for that connection."

As I think about how to proceed, I wonder: how do we shine some light onto Sinead's body and her experience of body in a way that doesn't injure, that doesn't demand she move in a certain direction? I am supportive of her intention to not be stopped by her body. Yet I also want to help her align with her body's power and intelligence to not be moved. It's this conflict that we need to resolve together.

The Immovable Body

"The other day," Sinead confides, "my older sister said, 'It isn't that you are so much bigger than other people who have gained weight. But you are so uncomfortable in your own body. You are so immovable and you are so stiff in the way you sit, the way you walk. And you've stopped communicating with your body. You used to have vivid facial expressions, but that's gone. I love you no matter what, but I can see the change, and it's painful for me to watch because I can see that you're unhappy with your own situation.'"

"I hear your sister wanting you to be more accommodating to her in the way you behave and move. She's against the stiffness. I'm imagining a response like, 'It's true. You're meeting a part of me that is not so movable. I've been too movable in my life, and that's beginning to surface, the beginning of experiencing myself as being stronger and less willing to bend. My body is showing you how that's emerging in me."

"That's right, that's absolutely right," Sinead says. "You nailed it. For so long I managed to hide it, to play that role very well, and now I can't do it anymore."

"She's loving, but it nonetheless shames the part of you that's stiffer. She's looking at it like it's a pathology, and not a part of what's birthing you into your next phase."

"You're absolutely right. Even today she said on the phone, 'I feel so sad after seeing you,' and I said, 'I'm sorry about that, but what am I going to do with your sadness and your worries? I don't need that.'"

"Good for you. I'd say, 'Dear Sister, this stiffness is needed. At one point I would have changed my outer composure and face to end your sadness. But that would sidetrack me from my journey. You didn't expect my healing to look like a person who's more immovable, you expected it to look like a more happy, easygoing person, a lighter person as opposed to a heavier person. You have an idea of healing that is too narrow.'"

"Yes," Sinead says, "more like conventional beauty."

"Right. The good part about your conversation with your sister is that it pushes you to focus more on your body. The negative part is the shame that came along with it. That's why I'm standing up for your stiffness and your body at the moment, because if we're going to address the body, we have to start by deeply respecting its stiffness, its size, its weight. We may be able to take another step, but first we have to say to the body, 'Before we try to change you into a flexible, happier, lighter being, I want you to know that I'm going to listen to you, get to know you, show respect for you and not treat you like you're a problem. You may be not the problem, you may be the medicine. Then maybe we'll think about bending, making it easier to meet people if you want to. First, though, I want to listen to you.'"

She is silent, thoughtful for a moment. Then she speaks.

"It was after the priest violated my body—that's when I began yo-yo dieting. I would either be unhealthily skinny, or put on extra weight. I went back and forth, and neither of them were very friendly, so to speak. When I was skinny, my ribs stuck out and I looked like someone who had been in a camp for far too long. I loved my bones. I was in love with feeling all those bones in my body."

"Wow. That's an amazing statement."

"And I thought, 'I have to get even thinner than this.' Of course, I got negative feedback, but I felt amazing, I felt beautiful even if I looked awful. I was vanishing. And when I gained weight, it was like a protection, like some stuffing that also protected me. The two states served similar purposes, had some qualities in common."

Disappearing into thinness or growing into protection:
both might serve the same purpose.

"Sinead, I've never heard somebody describe that as clearly and concisely, as eloquently as you just did—the beauty of vanishing in a hostile world where being visible would feel brutal, and then with gaining weight, the powerful protection of having a larger body."

"Thank you. I would eavesdrop on family members and friends and others saying, 'I can't stand to look at Sinead. She looks so sick, it makes me sick. It makes me feel bad to look at her.' And I thought, 'Wow. I am moving them away from me, they won't look at me. I have really succeeded.' I had become invisible and I was in charge of my own body."

"They saw the thin body that they didn't like," I reply, "and what they didn't see was the violence that happened before that. I want to say to your body, 'You've given me information, you've told me about vanishing. I'm hearing about the protection. I want to know more about your message and your intelligence there. You're telling me about the violation and its connections. And we can take time to learn about that so we can hold you as you ought to be held, in the proper love and respect, so we can see that there's a freedom for the body to become lighter, for you to make more movements, or not.'"

"Yes," Sinead says, "I want to feel lighter and become more flexible, but I also feel a part of me that's rock solid. It keeps me away from being seen because I know what will meet me: the shaming."

"Yes. So much ignorance, meanness, violence. So many shaming people who don't know how to look at a body and see beauty or power, who don't know how to look at a body and hear a story. How can you step out into such a violent world? People say overtly mean things, there's that too, but then there are people who will say, 'What happened to you, you used to be pretty?' or whatever. And so one way of giving you an immune system to protect you from those forces in the world is to have an inner immune system that sees you properly. The violence will come from the outside. There's no way we can prevent all of that from happening. But we can build a deeper view, a more genuine view, a non-shaming view. We can build that inside you so you can recognize ignorance more easily and ingest it less."

"Yes, there are things I would never participate in. I would never go to a bar and just hang out, that's not me. But there are small things that I would maybe love to do. Maybe meet people I know online in person. I would like for my body not to stop me from doing that."

"Something very strong inside you wants the freedom to go out and something even stronger, or just as strong, is not movable, doesn't want to be seen, needs to be protected. Won't even walk down the driveway. We've been exploring that immovability in different ways. It's possible, Sinead, that you can integrate some of the strength, the conviction, the power in that immovability. And it will help give you more freedom, because if you're told going out means you have to let go of what your deep body knowledge and self-love regarding your story manifests as—immobility—it probably won't work."

This is generally true. If a person wants to lose weight without integrating the intelligence and message the body holds in becoming larger, it ends up working against that intelligence, shaming that intelligence. It becomes a fight against one's body, a fight that will be near impossible to win.

I decide to work somatically, to deepen the inquiry into her body's intelligence.

"Let's take a moment to make contact with that strength,

to feel it your body. Is it in the stiffness of your body? The hardness in your back?"

"The stiffness in my body. Closing my mouth very hard. There's stiffness and pain in my jaw."

"Feel the stiffness of your jaw and express that same stiffness with your hand. Let it grip as tightly as your jaw, tighter, so your jaw doesn't hurt. Dear jaw, dear mouth, teach Sinead's hand to grip, to close, to tighten that way."

"Yes."

I use this technique of transferring a somatic experience into a hand expression in order to relieve the body of its pain, and so that the person can see and show what is happening inside.

"Now make your eyes look out through the eyes of the tightness, feel the tightness in your hand, look out through those eyes of tightness. Study that person, forget about Sinead as that soft person, be only her for the next minute."

"Yes."

Sinead is shape-shifting into her inflexible immovable self.

"Dear stiff person, we don't think you're only stiff, we think you have a message, intelligence, capabilities, powers."

"I am extremely strong. And I am stubborn beyond words. And I am the master of closing doors."

"Wow. What does that mean?"

"It means to close and shut the doors completely. To let nobody inside and to let nobody outside. I control the openings, and I control that freedom, and my strength must not be misjudged."

"That's you, Sinead. Claim that. Own that. The person who owns that will have more freedom to leave her house. You cannot leave without that power. You must not try to go outside without that. So if someone says an unkind word, or gives you an offensive glance or gesture, you can close that door right then and there. You get to choose that."

It blew me away to see this heroic aspect of Sinead—shamed as "stiff," fought against as being too heavy—come forward and so elegantly state its purpose, intelligence, capabilities, powers. There was no dithering, no people-pleasing. It is the antidote many women need in order to preserve and foster their own strength and agency in a world that expects them to be—often fatally—accommodating.

I learned later that the clergyman who molested and raped Sinead had locked his office door, preventing her from leaving. Psychologically speaking, he took the key from her—a key she needed to reclaim, a key that ought to be in her hands only.

Sinead's Success

Sinead's unfolding only led her to go out of her house a little more. That turned out to not be the most important direction her journey would take. Instead, she went further into herself, her true feelings, her sense of social justice and outrage about abuse, especially at the hands of the Church (which she expressed in her public writing), and her hunger to study depth psychology. Her spiritual life blossomed; her social voice blossomed. Although many would see her success as her achieving more conventional goals, I could readily see that she had become one of the most authentic people I have ever known.

Chapter Seventeen

Keisha: *Living Large*

*"You didn't come here to be somebody's doormat. You know deep
down who you are. You made this decision to play small because
you think it's safe or whatever, and you have to let that go."*

O VER THE COURSE of writing this book, I often wondered:
What would it look like for a woman *not* to grow up within
a society that shames little girls and takes away their ability to
feel good in their bodies, creating a lifetime of struggle? What
kind of woman would that little girl grow up to be?

I first encountered Keisha on Facebook, when she chimed
in on my public posts calling out men and white people for their
abuse of privilege and refusal to acknowledge their roles in systemic sexism and racism. I noticed she was a woman of color who
dressed boldly, which corresponded to the way she expressed
herself in words. I thought she might provide a valuable perspective to this book and was grateful when she agreed to be interviewed.

Keisha is an assistant principal in New York City and a dance
teacher. She's also certified in leading a moving meditation practice called FEM, which focuses on reclaiming the power of the
feminine, and holds an advanced certification in crystal healing.

She first shares about how she enjoys the way FEM provides
a safe space for sensual movement. "Under patriarchy, there's a

way sensuality becomes a very bad thing, because it means that you're either asking for something or being manipulative, instead of it just being part of how humans operate in the world. So many things are sensual. It's natural to explore all of your senses, and to breathe in flowers and experience the light from that. But patriarchy, because it has had this need to control women, has really tamped down on that and made people afraid."

This is just the first example of Keisha's inclination to experience life fully, unrestricted by oppressive, conventional belief systems. I was to learn that, for Keisha, life is not a problem to be fixed, an illness to be healed, but a celebration. When life is not a problem, shame evaporates.

"Yes, it's a patriarchal system that's also internalized," I say. "Energies, voices, belief systems, all of which want to control you as a woman, and me too as a man."

"A strong masculine is also essential," Keisha says. "You need decisiveness. You need the ability to protect others, right? We all need that, so the masculine is also divine, but the way that it gets expressed in patriarchy is sometimes quite toxic and sometimes very counterproductive. It's not sacred masculinity. I'm not someone who's thinking, saying that 'Oh, everything should be feminine.' Absolutely not, because nothing would get done, you know?" She laughs.

Keisha differed from all the other women I'd interviewed because she not only felt comfortable moving and embracing her embodied sensuality, she taught others to do the same. I could have noticed this and availed myself of her wisdom in this area right away, but I was still too caught up in the scope of my book and in my role as interviewer and educator. Every time I moved to be helpful, instructive, or psychological in my intent, the interview lost energy and Keisha took us in a different direction. I was soon to learn that it was I who was the student, Keisha the teacher and guide.

Keisha the Teacher

"What I'm wanting to explore with you or learn from you," I begin, "is about body size, body weight, body shame, and eating —wherever we go with that."

"I come from a family that is actually quite wonderful in some ways," Keisha answers. "Very colorful and creative people. My dad is a very successful jazz musician. But there's definitely a thread of addiction in my family. Along with the creativity and vibrancy, there's a very strong thread of melancholy, some very deep ancestral sorrow. Life for many people is quite challenging. I don't know if that's because that's the way it needs to be, but that is the way, at least in American culture, we have set things up. So many people have some kind of coping mechanism that helps them get through the day. In my household, people had addictions, so it wasn't surprising that I would develop a food addiction because I really didn't have the support that I needed. And I also grew up in a family that created some of the things that made me quite vulnerable in this world."

"So you found yourself eating more and becoming bigger because you considered it to be a way to cope with life's difficulties?"

"Yes, but I want to clarify that even though plenty of times I've wished to be smaller, more fit, stronger, and more flexible, I never felt that I wasn't pretty."

I thought that a door had opened to her childhood difficulties, patterns, and traumas, a door that I could help her walk through so we could uncover more of her psychology. But she responded, as at other times, with a "Yes, but," showing me that even those stories were not symptoms to resolve. She felt pretty; something in her was untouched, her relationship with her body was intact. I was still learning.

"That's wonderful," I say. "You may be the first woman I've met who feels that way, or admits it."

"I am of African heritage. Because of white supremacy, a lot of our aesthetics have shifted, but not all of them have. And so some of the aesthetics, like valuing thinness, just haven't been significant to me. I never felt that I wasn't sexy. I developed early, so all my life I've had this kind of validation, and even now, at fifty-eight, I still, when I walk down the street, I definitely get a lot of attention. Here in New York, it's not like in other parts of the country." She laughs. "They're saying something to you as you walk by."

"I hear you saying that your viewpoint is made up of your own sexiness, and New York street culture, and your experiences, and also, it's made up of your African heritage sensibilities."

"Yes. I think in the African American community, it's only been quite recent that there's been stigma around weight," Keisha says. "I didn't grow up in a culture where larger people were stigmatized. At least if they were, I was not aware of it. I remember how much big legs were admired. My dad had this girlfriend, and she used to talk about how she would wear things to make her legs look bigger, and I can remember people always telling me that I had big, pretty legs. And not just men. One time I was in my middle to late thirties, rollerblading. As I took off my rollerblades, these two African American women stopped to talk to each other about how pretty my big legs were."

Could you imagine if all girls were complimented by other women for having a big body? That would be a revolution.

"So you walk through the world feeling good about your body, all the time."

"Almost," she responds. "Sometimes I feel like in certain circles, if I act like I'm really proud of myself, people are going to be like, 'Who does she think she is?'"

She is teaching me that women aren't just shamed for their appearance. They're also shamed when they celebrate their bodies with pride.

"What kind of circles?"

"Mainstream circles, white circles. When white women receive compliments, they often diffuse it in some way. 'Oh, no, thank you. Oh, this old thing?' You know, like, 'I only paid $2 for this.' And then if you don't do that, people will get mad at you."

"And if you're not trying to conform to that expectation, how would you respond?" I ask.

"If someone complimented me on something, I would say, 'Oh, thank you. Yes, it's true.' But I don't think the world is ready for that."

My mind goes on dreaming of a world that is ready for women to walk through it, proud of their bodies and bodily expression.

Because Keisha grew up outside the white American culture, she can very clearly see and call out what might be subconscious to white women, that they're not allowed to think they are attractive. They can't openheartedly accept compliments without fear of blowback. This is like an external undertow that diminishes healing, pulling women away from self-love and toward shame.

"So if I were to say, 'Wow, you look beautiful today. I love your dress, I love your glasses,' or whatever, it would be radical for you to respond, 'Thank you, it's true. I love my body, I love my glasses, I feel really great today.' It challenges this oppressive paradigm for a woman, and especially a woman of color, to say, 'Yeah, I'm proud of myself. I like it. Thanks for the compliment. You're really right. I'm kind of a special, beautiful being here.'"

"Right. This is starting to shift. For example, think about how much people have embraced Lizzo [who just won a 2020 Grammy]. But when I was in my twenties, being liked by people was a lot more important to me. Of course, I'm human, I like to be liked. But now it's much more important to me that I am myself, the best self I can be, and I understand that some people will not like me for that, and it's not my job to take care of them. They have to figure it out for themselves. Now I'm really showing myself. I like to dress a certain way. I have a very, sort of very subtle but definitely provocative style. That is just my style. It's very easy to see that I put a lot of care into the way I dress. The way that the colors go together, the way that the patterns line up, it's obvious that I'm treating myself like I'm adorning myself. So, for example, some women at work really don't like me because they just feel like if I better matched the type of women that they see in magazines or in the media, then they would give me a pass. They're coming from a place of being in competition with each other for male attention, but if I looked thin and light-skinned, they would accept it more easily because that's the way that this hierarchy works."

Keisha's relationship with women's competitiveness for the male gaze and the privileges that might afford is also an enlightened one. She stands outside of it, watching it create a dance of pain.

"And those women, would they be thin and white?" I ask.

"They might not necessarily be white, but because white supremacy is still at work, they would be thinner and lighter skinned. I'm not saying that those other women are more or less beautiful, but I'm saying that I have my own beauty, and I really do feel that that is part of my work to really take a stand for my own beauty, whether or not it gets reflected back to me. Right?" Again, she had the answer, an answer so obvious but rarely lived—to stand for one's own beauty breaks down the competitiveness between women, disempowers the patriarchal gaze that creates the competitiveness in the first place."

"Absolutely!" I say. "That's amazing."

"I might not be in a world that is going to see beauty in people that are in the form that I'm in, and that's sad. But it's just like in China, back when they used to bind women's feet. People thought that was a good idea. Just because a lot of people think a certain way doesn't make it right. A lot of people have decided that broad noses are not attractive, that only noses that are more angular are attractive. The world could agree to that, but I'm not going to go along with it."

"I love what you're saying, I'm totally following you. You live in a world that has a viewpoint that you could collude with if you didn't have enough personal power. Hearing 'You shouldn't be as big, you should have a different nose, you should be lighter skinned, you shouldn't be so curvy, you certainly shouldn't show it off or enjoy a compliment.' That has an impact on a human being, right?"

"Right, yeah."

"What was it like for you when you didn't have this resiliency, that self-love?"

"Some of the stuff that people believe about black women is the most idiotic bullshit I've ever heard. But I have to navigate everything coming at me, because if I really resist it, in a very vigorous and adamant way, then I'm dismissed as the stereotype of an angry black woman. I always have to figure out *how can I be soft?* I just find that a lot of times it's more effective when I'm less direct, when I can kind of drop little crumbs for people to follow, rather than state things."

Keisha echoes a problem that many people of color are painfully aware of. While they are in situations where they have more awareness, wisdom, and understanding, they will suffer assaultive projections if they act accordingly. If they stand overtly in the role of teacher, momentarily superior in their understanding, the unconscious privilege of assuming one's own superiority, endemic in the white world, gets challenged and quickly acts out in resistance, as if to say, "How dare you act superior to me? I am superior to you."

Keisha's Counsel to
Women Who Want to Lose Weight

"Was there ever a period where you wanted to be thinner?"

"There was a time in my life when I lost ninety pounds, and I did that by rollerblading everywhere. It's not that I'm opposed to being thinner, but I believe that I'm beautiful in different ways, at any size. Over the past two years I've lost sixty pounds, but it's really been by retraining my brain. I've been using a model of thought: There's a circumstance, and the circumstance is always neutral, but you have a thought about that circumstance, and that thought leads to a feeling, the feeling leads to an action, and the action leads to a result. If I have a distressing thought about a circumstance, I might take the action of comforting myself with food I would not otherwise eat. And that action leads to a result of gaining weight. So I've really been looking at my thinking. How can I think about this differently?

And doing that helped me to eliminate certain things from my diet on a fairly regular basis. I avoid sugar and flour, although I do have one off-protocol meal a week. It's a slow process because I'm not doing anything radical, but I am eating in a more mindful way."

I decide to try to role-play with Keisha, but not because I am trying to help her have a breakthrough. She's had the breakthroughs long before we met. I want to learn from her more deeply and offer her teaching to others who would hopefully read her story.

"If I were a woman who came to you and said, 'I want to lose weight,' what would you say to me? Let's assume that I may just be not liking myself, and you were free to educate me, critically think with me."

"If you were a very close friend of mine and I suspected there were other things going on there, I would ask you, 'Why?' If you told me it was related to health, then I would really try to figure out how we could make this happen. If you told me, 'Well, I just don't like myself,' I would ask you to look at your thoughts. What makes you not like yourself?"

I answer, "I think I'm too big, and people don't like me, they don't hold doors for me and stuff like that."

"Okay," Keisha says, "So then I would ask you to consider, how are you holding yourself when you meet other people? People take the cue from you, right? So how are you signaling to people?"

"Well, I kind of cower. I'm shy, I dress neutrally so people don't notice me."

"What if we were to go out shopping and get you some clothes that you feel good in, that you feel powerful in, that you feel on top of the world in? It has to feel good on you, you have to really like the colors. We want to try to make this a very sensual experience. We want to try to bring in as many senses as we can."

"That's too scary for me. Maybe after I lose thirty pounds, then we'll go shopping."

"Well, you know what the funny thing is? People take their cues from you. So if you don't feel good about yourself, you could weigh ninety-eight pounds and you would have the same reactions from people."

"Wow, I love that. I love that. Thanks for doing that with me. I love the lesson that you're teaching."

"You have to love yourself as you are now. We are so incredible. We have so many options. You do get to change your body. You can change your look, your hair color. You can do so many things, but you have to love yourself as you are right now, and even as you're planning for those changes."

"There's a flavor, Keisha, to the way I'm hearing you talk about loving yourself that I don't always hear. Some people think that love doesn't look like going and getting the red dress. They think it's something else."

"Part of it is inviting more pleasure into your life. If you're a very sensual person, texture might be important to you. You need to have things that you really feel good in, that move well with you. Also, I really love the incredible diversity in our species. Some people love roses. They love that roses can be different colors. Some have thorns, some have very strong, vibrant smells, some have just like a little delicate whiff of fragrance. I feel that way about our species. I feel that we're really incredible because we have amazing diversity."

"What would you say to a woman who asks, 'How long will it take me to get to have that freedom? How long did it take you to get that?'"

"You have to be willing to let go of something."

"What do I have to let go of?"

"Of playing small. Because there's a part of you that knows the truth about you. You came to this planet. You decided to incarnate. You have a purpose. You came here for a reason. You didn't come here to be somebody's doormat. So you know deep down who you are. You just made this decision to play small because you think it's safe or whatever, and you have to let that go."

This is the essence of Keisha's freedom and wisdom. It's one part psychological, "Don't play small," and one part spiritual, "You came here for a reason." It's the seamless blending of these depths that flows through her movement, her dress, her words, and her relationship with herself.

"Ah, that's a big thing. What if I've learned to play small because of hurtful encounters and criticism?"

"Make the decision that these hurtful, critical people don't get to have space in your mind. It's just a habit to keep thinking that way. Our brains are quite lazy. They like to keep going around with the same thoughts over and over again. Whenever you want to have a new thought, to bring the new thought in a new direction, you have to practice it. So you have this idea that somebody gave you and it was misinformation, because it's not the truth. But your brain just wants to keep holding onto it, and so you have to retrain your brain. You have to say, 'That's not true,' every time you start to think that way. And decide, 'What are the thoughts I'm going to replace it with?'"

I must admit, I usually don't trust ideas like this. Too often, when people have unresolved hurts and traumas, trying to change their thoughts serves only to bypass, even dismiss, their wounds and stories. But Keisha was different. She knew her story. She was emotionally fluent regarding the perpetrations caused by family, sexism, and racism. Her path was about freedom, not healing. Her path was pride and joy. Her path was celebration. Her path was a teacher who modeled self-love.

"I would add," she says, "that I really believe in joy and playfulness. I believe that they're powerful weapons in the fight against all the different ways that we as humans oppress each other. If you can bring playfulness and joy into your life, what happens is sometimes you can change other people because they want some of what you're having. They want that lightness. They want that playfulness. They get attracted to that, and sometimes you can use that to shift their thinking, to open things up. So that's why I think it's a very powerful weapon."

"That's deep," I say. "I see that glow of the teacher in you. The deep one, not just, 'I want to teach you a new thought.' That's good, too. But more like 'I want to show you, I want you to touch it, I want you to hug it, I want you to feel it, I want you to know it. I want to change the way you think. I want to change the way you inhabit your skin and body.'"

I relate to that very deeply because that is at the heart of my intention with this book. I've been so blessed to encounter Keisha, and notice how much she lives these principles.

"Keisha, I just want to thank you so much for sharing so much with me—your celebration of yourself, of life, of the diversity of life, sensuality, joy. I hear that message."

"Oh, you're so very welcome. And I really want to thank you too. I love your posts. I often repost them because they're so eloquent and really nuanced. It's almost like you're this detective, but a detective of so many things. A detective of the heart, a detective of the human spirit, a detective of language, so that you really are able to tie together sometimes some things that seem quite separate but are actually very connected in sometimes insidious ways. I really thank you for the work that you're doing. I see the responses to things that you post, and I see that you're getting people to shift in their thinking."

Keisha's Biggest Lesson

Dear reader, you might be thinking, "This guy is really full of himself, including Keisha's praise in his book like this." I thought about that too, and almost deleted it. But that's Keisha's biggest lesson. Be beautifully, honestly, happily full of yourself. Then you won't need to find other, more socially sanctioned yet self-harming things to make you feel full.

I'm ending with Keisha's story because she flipped my script. She pulled the rug out from under my identity as teacher, healer, guide. And, as I reflect on the other stories, somehow they all seem to be less about psychological lessons and more about the beauty, sanctity, holiness of each of our paths.

We each sit on a kind of meditation cushion in our lives. Some sit on the cushion of physical illness, wrestling with body pains and limits as they do their part. Some sit on the cushion of relationship difficulties, seeking the right person, working out old patterns with friends and partners, learning to stay, or learning to leave. Some sit on the cushion of difficult feelings— depressions, anxieties, or rages—that won't let go, and disturb the flow of all they experience. But many sit on the cushion of body shame—eating, fasting, weighing, hiding, dieting, bingeing. For some, this is something they can "fix"; they can get over this struggle. But for the majority of women who have this problem in their path, whose life bids them to sit on this cushion, it's a lifelong struggle.

Once you see it as your meditation cushion, it transforms

from being a free-floating something to get over or "heal away," and more a place where you discover your power, your beauty, your intelligence, your spiritual authority. Women's bodies—their sizes, shapes, hungers, and all—become the site of enlightenment.

In a world that marginalizes the feminine, her body, and its wisdom, Keisha's viewpoint models a wisdom we all need in order to come into balance, to learn to love ourselves and each other, to care for the great mother, our planet, our Earth.

NOTES

Preface

xxvi ...before you learn that only five percent of women are successful at sustainably losing weight: Todd F. Heatherton, Meg Striepe, Fary Mahamedi, and Alison E. Field, "A 10-Year Longitudinal Study of Body Weight, Dieting, and Eating Disorder Symptoms," *Journal of Abnormal Psychology* 106, no. 1 (1997): 117-125, accessed June 19, 2020, http:// citeseerx.ist.psu.edu/viewdoc/down load?doi=10.1.1.721.4426&rep=rep1&type=pdf.

xxvi ...before you learn that eighty-one percent of ten-year-old girls are dieting regardless of their BMI index: L. M. Mellin, S. Scully, and C. E. Irwin, *Disordered Eating Characteristics in Preadolescent girls.* Paper presented at the annual meeting of the American Dietetic Association, Las Vegas, NV (1986).

xxvi ...before you learn that ninety-seven percent of women have violent voices in their heads about their bodies: Shaun Dreisbach, "Shocking Body-Image News: 97% of Women Will Be Cruel to Their Bodies Today," *Glamour*, February 3, 2011, accessed June 19, 2020, https://www.glamour.com/story/shocking-body-image-news-97-percent-of-women-will-be-cruel-to-their-bodies-today.

xxvi ...before you learn that being overweight, even mildly obese, is not a health risk: Katherine M. Flegal, Brian K. Kit, Heather Orpana, et al, "Association of All-Cause Mortality With Overweight and Obesity Using Standard Body Mass Index Categories: A Systematic Review and Meta-analysis," *JAMA* 309, no. 1 (January 2, 2013): 71-82, accessed June 19, 2020, doi: 10.1001/jama.2012.113905.

xxvi ...before you learn that the diet industry amasses over $70 billion: *The U.S. Weight Loss & Diet Control Market* (Tampa: Marketdata LLC, 2019), accessed June 19, 2020, https://www.marketresearch.com/Marketdata-Enterprises-Inc-v416/Weight-Loss-Diet-Control-12225125/?progid=91444.

Introduction

xxxi Of the people who go on a diet, ninety to ninety-five percent either stay the same weight or gain weight: "Methods for Voluntary Weight Loss and Control," National Institutes of Health Technology Assessment Conference Panel. *Annals of Internal Medicine* 199 (1993): 764-770.

xxxv **Less than five percent—some say eight or ten percent—of people are successful at losing weight and keeping it off:** Todd F. Heatherton, Meg Striepe, Fary Mahamedi, and Alison E. Field, "A 10-Year Longitudinal Study of Body Weight, Dieting, and Eating Disorder Symptoms," *Journal of Abnormal Psychology* 106, no. 1 (1997): 117-125, accessed June 19, 2020, http://citeseerx.ist.psu.edu/viewdoc/download?doi=10.1.1.721.4426&rep=rep1&type=pdf.

xliv **A major study showed that being overweight or mildly obese does not pose health risks:** Katherine M. Flegal, Brian K. Kit, Heather Orpana, et al, "Association of All-Cause Mortality With Overweight and Obesity Using Standard Body Mass Index Categories: A Systematic Review and Meta-analysis," *JAMA* 309, no. 1 (January 2, 2013): 71-82, accessed June 19, 2020, doi: 10.1001/jama.2012.113905.

xliv **However, research does show that gaining and losing weight:** Glenn A. Gaesser, *Big Fat Lies: The Truth About your Weight and Your Health* (New York: Fawcett Columbine, 2002).

lxi **In W.E.B. Du Bois's 1903 book:** W.E.B. Du Bois, *The Souls of Black Folk* (Chicago: A. C. McClurg & Co., 1903).

lxiii **One study measured the frequency of certain phrases women used:** Steve Bearman, Neill Korobov, and Avril Thorne, "The Fabric of Internalized Sexism," *Journal of Integrated Social Sciences* 1, no. 1 (2009): 15-16, accessed June 19, 2020, http://www.jiss.org/documents/volume_1/issue_1/JISS_2009_1-1_10-47_Fabric_of_Internalized_Sexism.pdf.

lxiii **Seven out of eight Americans with eating disorders are women:** "Eating Disorder Statistics," South Carolina Department of Mental Health, accessed June 19, 2020, http://www.state.sc.us/dmh/anorexia/statistics.htm.

lxiii **Ninety-seven percent of all women have hateful voices in their heads about their bodies:** Shaun Dreisbach, "Shocking Body-Image News: 97% of Women Will Be Cruel to Their Bodies Today" *Glamour*, February 3, 2011, accessed June 19, 2020, https://www.glamour.com/story/shocking-body-image-news-97-percent-of-women-will-be-cruel-to-their-bodies-today.

9: Megan: A Cocoon of the Right Size

98   **It reminds me of the "double consciousness" W.E.B. Du Bois wrote about:** W.E.B. Du Bois, *The Souls of Black Folk* (Chicago: A. C. McClurg & Co., 1903).

105 **The dominant culture trains us to think we must lose weight to stop the criticism (and a $70 billion diet industry banks on this thinking):** *The U.S. Weight Loss & Diet Control Market* (Tampa: Marketdata LLC, 2019), accessed June 19, 2020, https://www.marketresearch.com/Marketdata-Enterprises-Inc-v416/Weight-Loss-Diet-Control-12225125/?progid=91444.

11: Jasmine: You Don't Hurt Things that Are Beautiful

125 As I write this chapter years later, I wonder whether Jasmine knew that African American women were twenty percent more likely to have asthma: "Asthma and African Americans," U.S. Department of Health and Human Services Office of Minority Health, accessed June 19, 2020, https://minorityhealth.hhs.gov/omh/browse. aspx?lvl= 4&lvlid=15.

Acknowledgments

~~~~~~

I TAKE THIS opportunity to thank Candace Walsh as a friend, as an ally to women, and as a source of intelligence, grace, and beauty that informed this project. Candace, an award-winning writer and seasoned developmental editor, worked with me on drafts of chapters, transcripts of the therapeutic interviews, and hours of dialogue between us to help craft a book that is more relatable, engaging, and focused than it would have been without her involvement. Much respect, dear Candace.

Philosopher Theodor Adorno aptly declared that "the need to let suffering speak is a condition of all truth." Accordingly, I am indebted to the truth shared with me by the women who participated in the research that underlies the foundation of this book. They offered up their suffering *and more* in the form of fury and tears, grief and shame, and the deep wisdom held in their hearts, minds, and bodies. Further, they agreed to being part of an honest conversation and education that would flow from the telling of their stories publicly. I labored for years in writing, editing, and reediting this book in order to honor the truth they shared with me.

In addition, countless women have shared similarly in private sessions and groups I facilitated on weight-loss, body shame, and sexism. As a man, I am obliged to honor all they taught me by educating others to the very best of my capacity.

Although I have many privileges in my life, some social, some personal, I could not have continued to learn, to write, to vision and revision this book without great winds of friendship at my back. Some friends were consistent and persistent in having that wind blow strong and at the right time. I am grateful for India Elaine Garnett, whose soul force was alchemized by America's ugly shadow of racism. Her noble grace and bright-star love never fades. Her wisened hands penned the book's foreword.

I also thank Catherine Hiesiger, who lifted me when I fell, time and time again, serenading me with song, carrying me in her heart; Shevanee Cardoza, who taught me to dream big and stand clearer in my authority; Carolyn Riker, who always believed in the power and intelligence of this work transmitted in the form of her poetry-soaked words; and Leonora Lorenzo, whose depth of embodied feeling upon reading the manuscript left me knowing the task of writing this book was indeed a calling. Thank you.

There were more than sixty people—psychologists, psychotherapists, and women who know, intimately, the power of the patriarchal gaze to foster body shame and self-hatred—who shared their viewpoints, their insights, their appreciations, their critiques, and their raw feelings upon reading the manuscript. Knowing how a book impacts readers was a bigger gift than I had realized. Actually, it was enormous.

Elder and teacher, Arnold Mindell, has guided me along my path for more than twenty-five years. The first time I sat with him, he asked, "David, are you writing?" "Only in my journals,"

I said. I didn't yet have the freedom to take my vocation as a writer more seriously. Since then I have written three books and authored more than one hundred articles and blog posts published in a variety of venues. Arny always dreamt a life for me that was one step further and bigger than my own eyes could see. That is a gift, without which I would not be here writing these acknowledgments.

Salome Schwarz has counseled and walked me through the twists and turns, the torments and glories, of my relationships, my inner life, and my career callings. Her profound faith in Spirit reminds me always that the life that I look forward to is the one I am already living.

Jeff Braucher, copy editor, took to each word, comma, and sentence with fine craft, care, and consideration. Thank you, Jeff, for your ready attention to my manuscript.

Lisa Blair, my partner, my best friend, my wife, touches everything I do with love's blessing. She treats every dream I have as she treats her garden—like a living soul worthy of the greatest care for its blossoming. Galway Kinnell wrote, "Sometimes it is necessary to reteach a thing its loveliness" so that it may flower. I, and all I feel, think, and do, have flowered because her true and most tender hands have bestowed this "reteaching" upon me.

One morning, reading the feedback of dozens of women who were reading the book, Lisa and I noted how many spoke of their tears, anger, sleepless nights, as well as their painful and powerful memories. Lisa said, "Give me a half hour, I have an idea for the book cover." I had been wrestling with different titles and used professional cover designers in the past, but when I saw what she proposed, I said, "That's it." In retrospect, I am not surprised that she "saw" the face of the book.

About the Author

D AVID BEDRICK, J.D., DIPL. PW, grew up in a family marked by violence. While his father's brutality was clear—belts, fists, and harsh words—his mother's denial and dismissal of the violence had its own more covert power. He came away with a life dictum: people need to be believed. That belief was not only literal—what a person says is matched by some objective observation—but also psychological: what a person experiences and how they behave, however subjective or seemingly irrational, are worthy of being viewed as if they were carrying sacred messages.

Speaking from this dictum at an early age provoked criticisms from each of his parents. His father called him a "dreamer," meaning out of touch and unrealistic. His mother told him, "You can't change the world."

Fortunately, these efforts to censure him landed in the right spot. David spent more than twenty-five years studying Jungian psychology and nighttime dreams. He pursued an education in conflict resolution focused on world problems (e.g., race, gender, wealth inequality, anti-Semitism) and eventually went to law school hoping to "change the world." Graduating at the top his class, he began helping women and children in the midst of the family violence inherent in domestic abuse, divorce, and custody disputes.

David's initial foray into wanting to understand family and social dynamics led him to study organizational psychology at the University of Minnesota. That training formed the basis of a twelve-year effort into changing the world by transforming institutions. He consulted to and trained managers in 3M, Honeywell, United Way, the U.S. Navy, and dozens more.

Thirsty for more potent transformative skills, he left Applied Personnel Technologies, the consulting firm he co-founded, and pursued clinical training in working with individuals and large-scale conflict at the Process Work Institute (an offshoot of the Jung Institute). He became a teacher and adjunct faculty member at the Process Work Institute and later at the sister institute in Warsaw, Poland, where he taught about the intimate link between the body and the psyche. Still on the faculty, he is also a member of the Institute's ethics committee.

David's passion for teaching, changing minds and hearts, led him to becoming an adjunct faculty member at the University of Phoenix for eight years, where he taught courses in human services (from Clinical Interviewing, to Addictions and Diversity), philosophy (Critical Thinking and Ethics), and conflict resolution in their master's program in business. It was there that he began his study of body shame and eating when woman after woman presented their final papers in Critical Thinking on their personal struggles. David started a research project with twenty-one women who gave him permission to record several sessions on the issue. His findings broke the mold, particularly how shame and self-hatred not only motivated many women to diet, but prevented them from succeeding at their goal.

One day he was watching a Dr. Phil episode where women were presenting their struggles with weight loss. Dr. Phil tried to motivate the women by showing them their own wedding dresses modeled by women who were thinner. Aghast, David began writing down the details of Dr. Phil's approach and how that caused the shame and lack of success he discovered in his research. This became a significant section of his book *Talking Back to Dr. Phil*, which also included sections on other topics, from family violence to issues of addiction and power. Professor, poet, writer, and activist Nikki Giovanni, winner of an unprecedented seven NAACP Image Awards, wrote, "At last someone is taking on Dr. Phil with good sense and great humor. Good for Mr. Bedrick to decide to pull off the gloves and have an emotional slugfest with an over-the-high-school bully. *Talking Back to Dr. Phil* is a must-read."

And acclaimed experts and best-selling authors in the field of women's body shame and weight loss, Jane R. Hirschmann and Carol H. Munter, wrote, "David Bedrick understands that real change or transformation requires challenging accepted dogma and then approaching problems with compassion and curiosity. A great advocate for stopping the madness of body hatred and dieting."

Realizing that his message was too radical for a university curriculum, David moved to Santa Fe, New Mexico, to begin the formation of what is now the Santa Fe Institute for Shame-Based Studies, which offers classes on shame and trauma as well as body shame and weight loss.

Along the way, he wrote his second book, *Revisioning Activism*, which includes essays on sexism, body shame, and eating, as well as discussions about psychology's role in social activism. *Foreword Reviews* wrote, "David Bedrick's *Revisioning Activism* seeks to right individual and social wrongs through writing. This wide-ranging collection examines topics like racism, weight loss, and women's self-esteem, as well as current events, and how Process Psychology can be applied within individual lives. General readers will find comfort in these practical essays that offer hope for those who believe they must suffer silently and alone, while therapists will have their methodologies reaffirmed or challenged." *Revisioning Activism* was awarded *Foreword Review*'s 2016 INDIES Finalist designation.

David has also written blog posts for *Huffington Post* and *Psychology Today* on the topic, and been interviewed on more than thirty radio shows, including New Dimensions Radio. *Psychology Today* has published eighty-five of his posts, which have now been read by more than two million people.

David's initial research on the effects of body shame on weight-loss efforts, esteem, and personal empowerment is now sixteen years old and as relevant as ever. While body shame is perhaps the greatest pain and derailer at the root of almost all weight-loss efforts, its impact is almost never mentioned in conventional thinking and strategies. Sexism, a significant part of the creation of body shame in women, is also almost never mentioned. Talking to women about their bodies without talking about personal and social shaming is a conversation stripped of deep truth, true power, and a path to a sustainable self-love.

It is the absence of this truth, its veritable denial, which resonated with David's childhood story and dictum to believe people. *You Can't Judge a Body by Its Cover* is an expression and agent of that belief.